Access to Ambulatory Care and the U.S. Economy

Access to Ambulatory Care and the U.S. Economy

Frank A. Sloan
Vanderbilt University

Judith D. Bentkover
Arthur D. Little, Inc.

Lexington Books
D.C. Heath and Company
Lexington, Massachusetts
Toronto

Library of Congress Cataloging in Publication Data

Sloan, Frank A
  Access to ambulatory care and the U.S. economy.

  Includes index.
  1. Physician services utilization—Economic aspects—United States.
2. Ambulatory medical care—United States—Utilization. 3. Poor—Medical
care—United States. 4. Unemployed—Medical care—United States.
5. Inflation (Finance)—United States. 6. United States—Economic
conditions—1971-   I. Bentkover, Judith D. joint author. II. Title.
RA410.7.B46   362.1   78-19537
ISBN 0-669-02510-0

Published simultaneously in Canada.

Printed in the United States of America.

International Standard Book Number: 0-669-02510-0

Library of Congress Catalog Card Number: 78-19537

To our spouses, Paula and Stuart

Contents

List of Figure
and Tables

Foreword

Since the mid-1960s and continuing throughout the present decade, this nation has made an increasing budgetary commitment to the objective of improving access to health care for all Americans. At the same time, new government and private organizations have been established to monitor quality of care, plan the allocation of health resources, and promote efficiency in the provision of health care services. These initiatives have moved forward despite adverse economic conditions.

This study provides evidence that, despite the state of the economy, some gains in access to health services, attributable at least in part to public programs, have been made during the 1970s. Such findings are gratifying to someone who deals with these matters on a daily basis. Nevertheless, it is clear that many deficiencies in the health care system remain, and access is by no means universal. In addition to our internal evaluations, we in government must look to outsiders for evidence on the degree to which public programs live up to our original expectations.

Past research by economists specializing in health care issues has principally dealt with questions related to efficiency in the delivery of health care services, such as economies of scale in hospitals. More recent research includes such topics as manpower substitution in physicians' practices and hospitals, and there are several recent and ongoing evaluations of the effects of regulation on the health care sector. The propensity of economists to emphasize efficiency is understandable, not only because such issues have policy relevance, but also because the methodological tools of economics are more powerful in dealing with efficiency than with equity issues. But I admit to being somewhat perplexed as to why economists in such human resources fields as education have been concerned with who benefits from and who pays for education programs while health economists have largely neglected such issues in their research.

One of the contributions of the book by Frank Sloan and Judith Bentkover is their discussion of an economic approach toward assessing access to health care. Many of the variables evaluated by persons in other social science disciplines are also amenable to economic analysis, and economics has a definite contribution to make toward a better understanding of the behavior underlying various access measures.

The development of new public programs and the evaluation of existing ones ideally would incorporate knowledge gained from analysis of trends as well as more methodologically sophisticated inquiries. But often the lags between important developments, such as changes in economic circumstances, the reporting of statistical health care data, and the time required by analysts to assemble and communicate findings is too long to provide a useful input into the policy process. To wait for data and research findings would be to place a needless burden on those who might suffer the most. Fortunately, much has been and can be learned from past experience that can be applied to predict future changes. Although history may not precisely repeat itself, many behavioral forces remain unchanged.

This study reports many new findings of behavioral responses to economic and other forces and substantially enhances our understanding of factors that influence access to health services. In view of our commitment toward continual improvement of access, Professor Sloan and Dr. Bentkover have made a very timely contribution to the development of informed public policy in this area.

Karen Davis
Deputy Assistant Secretary
for Planning and Evaluation/Health
United States Department
of Health, Education, and Welfare

Acknowledgments

Several individuals have made substantial contributions to this study. This research was supported by the National Center for Health Services Research under a contract with Policy Analysis, Inc., Brookline, Massachusetts. Because of bureaucratic problems in obtaining Office of Management and Budget clearance for our survey instrument this was an unusually difficult project, both from the standpoint of the National Center and our research team. We thank Ira Raskin and James Daugherty, our project officers at the National Center for their assistance throughout this project. In particular, when OMB approval was not obtained in time to field our access survey because of a number of unanticipated bureaucratic obstacles fully beyond our control, both Dr. Raskin and Mr. Daugherty helped us restructure the project around secondary data bases.

Dr. Ronald Andersen and Dr. Lu Ann Aday of the Center for Health Administration Studies, University of Chicago, deserve special thanks for sharing their data from the Robert Wood Johnson Foundation sponsored Medical Access Study (MAS) for purposes of our research. Without the MAS data base, the failure to obtain OMB approval for our own survey would have meant the end of the project.

Roger Reynolds, a member of the Center for Health Administration Studies staff, provided valuable programming assistance on aspects of our research based on MAS data. He was far more than a programmer. He served as a colleague, giving valuable advice on econometric issues.

Arthur Sobel was the programmer on work involving the Health Interview Survey. His careful documentation made working at a distance (Nashville-Boston) possible. We thank Denise Boland, Ellen Boland, Anita Gibbs, and James Kanak for careful and painstaking compilation of tables.

Professor Ralph Berry spent many days on a draft of this report. Not only did he sharpen our discussion in several places, but he also helped improve the report's readability. There is, of course, only so much that even Professor Berry can do. We therefore remain responsible for the inadequacies that remain.

As we have noted, this has been a difficult project to administer because of the change in direction necessitated by the failure to obtain OMB clearance. James Boland and Mary Louise Fisher of Policy Analysis deserve our thanks for handling many of the administrative matters associated with this project.

On numerous occasions, we called Ethel Black at the National Center of Health Statistics for data and for clarification. She was always ready to help and thereby made the job of analysis in chapter 3 far easier.

Typing of drafts and the final manuscript were responsibilities shared by Freida Knight, Nancy Richardson, and Sylvia Haywood. Their dedication to the work, their responsiveness to the whims of the authors, their cheerfulness, and their pride taken in a job well done are all greatly appreciated.

Four unnamed reviewers read and commented on a draft of this report. We thank you for your valuable comments (whoever you are).

Introduction

Substantial public investments have been made during the past decade with the purpose of removing barriers patients have historically faced in obtaining health care services. The most important of these programs are Medicare and Medicaid on the financing side and government support of health professions education on the supply side. The rationale of these programs has been to improve access of the population to mainstream medicine.

By any number of criteria, the performance of the U.S. economy, especially in contrast to the 1960s, has been disappointing. During 1974-1975, the nation experienced one of the highest rates of inflation in its history and the most severe recession since the Great Depression. The effects of abnormally high inflation and unemployment are still being felt during the late 1970s. The impact of adverse economic conditions on health care costs has been documented.[1] The effects on patient access to care are much more subtle and less easily measured. The primary objective of this study is to gauge the impact of adverse economic conditions of the 1970s, especially the mid-1970s, on patient access to ambulatory care. Have the gains of the past decade been partially or fully reversed during the past few years by adverse conditions in the economy? And if so, have low income groups been predominantly affected?

Our emphasis is on ambulatory care for two reasons. The physician is the "gate-keeper" of the health care system. His advice and consent is needed before the patient is admitted to the hospital, receives care from specialized units, and is able to purchase numerous kinds of prescription drugs. Furthermore, there is currently rather widespread agreement that hospitals are, if anything, over-utilized. Such policies as certificate-of-need and utilization review are actually efforts to reduce the use of hospital services offering low potential marginal benefits. With the exception of surgery, there is at present far less concern about overutilization in the domain of physicians' services. In fact, in the area of primary or "first-contact" services, there is still substantial concern that several groups within the U.S. population may remain underserved.

A superficial answer to our question about recent trends in access to ambulatory care could be obtained rather easily. No single indicator for the U.S. population as a whole suggests a *dramatic* decline in access to physicians' services. Where decreases are evident, they are small. And some indicators actually show continued improvements. A superficial approach has two important shortcomings. First, important distributional effects can be easily obscured. If five or ten percent of the population experiences welfare losses, measures of the population as a whole may obscure this phenomenon. In fact, if the recent Canadian experience with universal health insurance, briefly reviewed in chapter 2, is any guide, gains or losses in the access on the part of the poor may coincide with the reverse experience—losses or gains in access— on the part of the more affluent. It is necessary to isolate and identify the experience of particular segments of the population. Second, inflation and recession are by no means the sole determinants of access. It is therefore inappropriate to attribute everything, as a superficial approach would have us do, to conditions prevailing in the economy during the mid-1970s. More in depth cross-tabular analysis and multivariate analysis is needed.

Expenditures for physician fees, within and outside the hospital, account for approximately one-fifth of health care spending. In 1976, 26.4 billion dollars was spent for physician services. In light of the ever-increasing allocation of resources to health care, is society reaping an adequate return compared to alternative uses of those resources? In order to answer this question we evaluate the evidence pertaining to the access to physician services. We attempt to study the factors affecting an individual's access to ambulatory care and draw inferences regarding the efficacy of further increases in national expenditures directed at improving the access to health care. In particular, we investigate the differential impact of an individual's demographic characteristics and an individual's economic environment.

A second purpose of this study is to advance the state of the art of research on access to ambulatory care. Only recently have social scientists become aware of some of the more important behavioral influences on access. Most of the dimensions of access are amenable to modeling efforts. Events do not "just happen" in this area any more than in other areas that have been the topics of theoretical and empirical inquiry for years. More basic or general research on access is not without potential payoffs for policy purposes. Thus, for example, this study provides new information on the effects of physician availability on various dimensions of access.

This study consists of a review of pertinent literature on patient access to ambulatory care, analysis of time series and cross-sectional evidence of a descriptive nature, and multivariate analysis. Both our descriptive and multivariate analysis is based on unpublished data from 1969–1975 Health Interview Surveys, conducted by the National Center for Health Statistics, and the Medical Access Study, conducted in 1975 by the Center for Health Administration Studies and the National Opinion Research Center, both affiliated with the University of Chicago.

Chapter 1 sets the stage for our analysis. Our concept of access is briefly discussed, notions to be expanded in chapter 2. We then review recent trends in inflation and unemployment and discuss the multidimensional effects of inflation and recession on household behavior.

Chapter 2 provides a literature review of pertinent studies on four dimensions of access: utilization of physicians' services; utilization relative to need for physicians' services; process measures; and indicators of patient satisfaction with care received. Although no previous studies have specifically assessed the impacts of inflation-recession, there are estimates of partial impacts of real patient income and health insurance coverage on various access indicators; and these estimates are clearly germane to our investigation. Results from prior work imply as a general matter that patient ability to pay is a factor in access. While the findings of past studies are important for the preceding reason, the review serves two other purposes. First, it provides a conceptual framework for much of the empirical analysis in the remaining chapters. Second, the results themselves permit comparison with findings from the Health Interview Survey and Medical Access Study presented for the first time in this study.

Chapter 3 presents a cross-tabular analysis and a multivariate analysis of time-series data from the 1969–1975 Health Interview Surveys. In these analyses, the entire emphasis is on utilization of physician services and this utilization relative to need. Attention is paid to utilization for the population as a whole and to various groups within the population, categorized by age, family size and income, and employment status.

Regression analysis is based on a time series of quarterly observations covering the years 1969–1975. We specify two equations. The first equation includes physician visit rates as the dependent variable; the second includes one of two alternative health status measures as the dependent variable—restricted-activity days and bed-disability days. The health status measures are employed, alternatively, as explanatory variables in our utilization regressions. In this way we are able to assess the direct impact of inflation and unemployment on utilization; these variables are also included as explanatory variables in our utilization regressions. We can also assess the indirect effects of inflation and unemployment on utilization. If deteriorating economic conditions affect health adversely, as previous research by Brenner[2] suggests, and poor health has a positive effect on utilization, inflation and recession have indirect effects on utilization operating via health status. The sum of direct and indirect effects are the total effects. The regression analysis is on balance quite fruitful and enables us to isolate effects of inflation-recession not evident from two-way tabulations.

While all the empirical chapters contain findings pertinent to the link between job loss and access, the major direct evidence on the impact of inflation on access is reported in chapter 3. Since expectations play such a prime role in the inflationary process, time-series analysis is particularly suitable for assessing the impact of inflation. The remaining chapters are based on cross-sectional data bases. Furthermore, only chapter 3 contains an assessment of response lags to changes in exogenous factors.

Data from the 1974 Health Interview Survey (HIS) are analyzed in chapter 4. This particular survey is especially useful for purposes of this study because 1974 was a bad year for the economy and a special supplement on access to health care services was conducted as part of the HIS in that year. In contrast to chapter 3, where utilization and utilization-need measures are emphasized, the focus in chapter 4 is on process and satisfaction with care measures.

The National Center for Health Statistics ensured that the tapes of individual responses to the 1974 HIS were available to us. Consequently, we are able to pose and derive answers to three basic questions in chapter 4. First, over the course of 1974, is there any indication that access to physicians' services deteriorated? Certainly the economy deteriorated substantially during 1974. Thus one could well expect access to be adversely affected and for the effect to be evident even over a short time period. Second, as of 1974, how did the employed and unemployed compare in terms of several dimensions of access? Third, how did the access of the short-term and the long-term unemployed compare? The 1974 HIS data base is unique among data sources containing access information in permitting one to distinguish among the unemployed according to the duration of their unemployment.

One of the more disturbing trends, evident from data presented in chapter 3 and from many published studies, is the growth in importance of hospital outpatient clinics and emergency rooms as the source of ambulatory care and services. Although these sites of care have a definite role to play within the health care system as a whole, they are thought to be inadequate in providing primary care services. Chapter 5 is exclusively devoted to the analysis of patient choice of site of care. If adverse economic conditions drive greater numbers of persons away from the office-based physicians, one can conclude that there is some evidence that access has indeed declined, even though this indicator, like the others, has definite limitations as an overall measure of access.

The data base for work in both chapters 5 and 6 is the Medical Access Study. In both chapters, we are principally concerned with six policy issues. First, how does the fact that the opportunity wage has fallen affect patients' choices? As noted above, on theoretical grounds, we expect employment status to affect the opportunity cost of consuming health care services in particular and consumption of all goods and services in general. Second, what role does family income play in patients' choices? For example, to what extent do individuals eschew hospital-based ambulatory services as their incomes rise? The public sector can affect the real income of various groups within the population by means of its tax-transfer policies. Third, how closely does private health insurance relate to various dimensions of access? Lee[3] has estimated that the loss of private group health insurance coincident with the loss of employment is substantial. If there is a definite link, there is reason to argue for proposed government programs that provide continued health insurance coverage to the unemployed. Fourth, the shortcomings of Medicaid as a means for assuring the poor access to "mainstream medicine" are, by and large, well documented. During recessions, larger numbers of persons become dependent on Medicaid. In both chapters 5 and 6, we gauge the experiences of Medicaid recipients in terms of various process dimensions of access. Fifth and sixth, we measure race-ethnicity and physician availability effects on access.

Whereas chapter 5 considers patient choice of site, which encompasses several elements of access simultaneously, chapter 6 examines three of the process dimensions explicitly: the time the patient spent after arrival waiting for the physician; the time the physician spent with the patient; and the delay between the time an appointment was made and the actual visit. As in chapter 5, the analysis is conducted with reference to a specific recent visit. The same explanatory variables and samples are used. The four samples, analyzed in both chapters, are: retirees ages 65 and over with both husband and wife present; female heads of household ages 25 to 64; married men, and married women, ages 25 to 64.

Chapter 7 presents concluding remarks. Implications of our findings for public policy are discussed.

A disadvantage of using surveys that were designed for other purposes is that some information one may need is missing. This is the case with the wage-income component of the models developed in chapters 5 and 6. In an appendix to this book, we have outlined how we derived our wage-income variables from the rather limited income information provided by the Medical Access Study. This discussion should be of interest to readers wanting more detail on the wage and income variables used in chapters 5 and 6. The appendix also includes new information on the economics of time.

Notes

1. U.S. Council on Wage and Price Stability, *The Problem of Rising Health Care Costs,* Washington: U.S. Printing Office, April 1976.

2. M. Harvey Brenner, *Estimating Social Costs of National Economic Policy: Implications for Mental and Physical Health and Criminal Aggression,* Washington: Joint Economic Committee of the U.S. Congress, 1976.

3. A. James Lee, *Employment, Unemployment, and Health Insurance,* Cambridge, Mass.: Abt Books, 1979.

Access to Ambulatory Care and the U.S. Economy

1 Background and Overview

Over the years, numerous instances have been documented of the difficulties patients encounter in obtaining access to health care services. Many arguments advanced by proponents of government programs in the health services field reflect an underlying concern with equity in the distribution of health care services, or at least the concern that all citizens receive a minimum level of these services.

During the 1960s and 1970s, governments at all levels have substantially increased outlays on programs having direct and indirect effects on access. The largest of these include Medicare and Medicaid and support for medical education. More recently, policies directed toward primary care have been implemented to address an allegedly inappropriate mix of services.

In spite of the enormous increase in the role of government, there is a widespread view that (1) important access barriers persist, and (2) these barriers affect the poor and, at least to some extent, the nonpoor. For example, as Professor Anne Somers has noted:

> A considerable part of the problem . . . is the fact that so many people still lack good access to health care. For many, it is quantitatively deficient. For many more, including many in middle and upper income categories, it is qualitatively lacking, particularly in the educational influence of a good doctor-patient relationship, a lack that probably disturbs the patient even more than it does the doctor.[1]

Although most writings on this subject emphasize that the current situation is far from ideal, the trends observed in several access indicators over the past fifteen years are encouraging on the whole.[2] This encouraging impression is confirmed by our study.

Trends are often inferred by making comparisons of data for years five or ten years apart. Such comparisons may obscure meaningful short-run patterns which, although seemingly temporary, may nevertheless elicit policy concern. The inflation-recession of the 1970s is a matter of considerable consequence in both the United States and in other countries. One certainly cannot rule out the possibility that economic conditions, such as inflation and recession, have dramatic effects on medical care consumption patterns without first examining the empirical evidence. The marked changes in both the inflation

1

and unemployment picture during the 1970s have been well publicized by the news media.

Until recently, economists viewed the consequences of inflation, at least in the U.S. context, as being primarily redistributional; the gains of some persons largely offset the losses of others. To the extent that this is so, one could ostensibly identify the gains and the losses and assess whether the transfer should be viewed as desirable or undesirable. There has been an increasing realization, however, that inflation has a real aggregate output effect as well as distributional effects. This means that inflation reduces the total amount of goods and services available for society as a whole, as well as affecting the distribution of those goods and services.[3]

By contrast, both the redistributional and real aggregate output effects of recession have long been recognized. Moreover, while there is still some room for debate as to how low-income families fare relative to high-income families during inflations, there is little doubt that lower income families bear a disproportionate share of the burden of recessions. It must be emphasized that each inflationary and recessionary period has unique as well as common causes, and therefore each has unique as well as common features. Certainly a unique feature of most such periods in the 1970s in particular is the presence of unusually high and concurrent rates of inflation and unemployment. Consequences of inflations and recessions also differ, depending on government responses to adverse economic conditions. For instance, whether inflation imposes a special burden on the poor and the aged depends in part whether transfer payments keep pace with the growth of prices.

Access Defined

The term "access to health care services" is used often, and it is subject to several interpretations. There is no reason to settle on a single definition. Given the large number of serious students of this subject, it would be presumptuous to do so. Yet it is essential to understand what the principal definitions are and what they imply.

A first group of access measures refers to *characteristics of the population and health care providers in a geographic area.* Included among these are: family income; health insurance coverage; and the number and distribution of health manpower and facilities in an area. On theoretical and empirical grounds, one may reason that health services use is likely to be lower among the economically disadvantaged and in areas with relatively few health resources. Federally designated "underserved areas," used for operating specific federal manpower programs, have these characteristics. For many purposes it may be useful to examine these patient and provider characteristics; given data limitations, it is sometimes necessary to make decisions on the basis of limited surrogates.

A second type of access measure relates to health services *utilization* in the aggregate and/or for certain population subgroups. A more refined but related measure is *utilization relative to an empirical indicator of need*, for example, restricted activity days, bed disability days. There are those who strongly support the use of utilization-need measures of access. For example, according to Andersen:

> "Equitable distribution" does not imply that everyone should receive the same amount of health services. Instead, I propose that an "equitable distribution" of health services is one in which illness (as defined by the patient and his family or by health care professionals) is the major determinant of the distribution. . . . Perceived need and evaluated need are the major determinants of health services use in such a system, because of the well-established relationships between health and age, sex and marital status. On the other hand, social structure, health beliefs, family resources, and community resources should have less impact on utilization. Inequity is suggested, for example, if the distribution of services is determined by race, income or availability of facilities. Empirically, a distribution of services may be defined as more equitable, the stronger the association between utilization, perceived and evaluated need and demographic variables on the one hand, and the weaker the association between utilization and social structure, health benefits, family resources and community resources on the other hand.[4]

Although this type of measure has many attractive features, and our empirical analysis includes an assessment of utilization-need, there are also problematical aspects. The most important of these involves the definition of need. Social science has established systematic variations in perceptions of need and in the ways that medical symptoms are presented according to measurable characteristics of persons and their environments. If, for instance, persons in a particular subculture are more likely to present themselves as "sick," the above definition would, holding other factors constant, in effect argue in favor of a redistribution toward that subculture.[5] Moreover, illness may sometimes be used to legitimize absences from work and school.[6] Attempts to achieve greater equity in the delivery of the health services may effectively subsidize absenteeism. Subsidies on this basis would violate other ethical principles held by many, such as that people be compensated on the basis of their contributions. These points also serve to emphasize that no one measure is likely to be fully consistent with the ethical principles held by most members of society.

Proponents of programs such as public education do not typically argue for equality in the use of educational services, whether measured in terms of years of schooling or in relation to some external measure, such as native intelligence. Minimum requirements on educational attainment are established under state statutes. But above these requirements, there is concern about the nature of the child's education, a qualitative dimension. There is also comparatively greater emphasis on components of the price facing the student—such as those associated with travel to the educational facility and foregone earnings—as well as direct out-of-pocket payments for books and tuition. These factors dominate concern for equality in use in the case of public education. In fact, substantial differentials in use, in the presence of a low price of education, are widely tolerated and even advocated by "liberals" in the field of education.

It seems reasonable to note one implication for health care delivery in this context. The use of such a standard as equality-in-use or even equality-in-use-relative-to-need, would not likely lead to a lack of public interest in distributional issues. One gets an indication of this from critics of the Medicaid program as the program is currently constituted. If Medicaid has raised the consumption of services by the poor in relative as well as absolute terms, it still has not eliminated such complaints as those dealing with the impersonal care received by the poor and the long waiting times experienced by the poor in clinics.

A third class of access measures encompasses *process indices*. By process, we mean descriptors of qualitative aspects of the patient's contact with the health care system: whether the patient has a usual source of care; travel time to the physician; waiting time in the physician's office; delays to an appointment; mean time that the physician and aides spend with the patient per visit; availability of the physician at night and on weekends. Thus defined, process measures influence utilization, but they too depend on a set of exogenous forces, some of which reflect the condition of the economy. Because they measure qualitative features of the patient experience, they merit study in their own right.

This study emphasizes process measures more than many other studies of access. However, it should be noted that these process measures have their critics. For example, Salkever, in arguing the superiority of a use-need measure of equity states that

> ... a norm based on these (process) characteristics might specify that travel times to primary care sources should be equal across population groups. But substantial divergences from this specification are not necessarily inconsistent with complete or almost complete equality of use.[7]

Salkever's point is correct *if* one accepts the premise that equality of use relative to some measure of need is of primary importance, but there are also counterarguments. Clearly, recent concern with "humaneness" in the context of health care delivery is primarily a concern about the nature of services received. There is comparatively less interest with the efficacy of health services in causing improvements in health status and with the lack of uniformity in visits to physicians in relationship to a measure of need. One might justify long waiting time in clinics and physicians' offices, especially on the part of the poor, in terms of economic efficiency. The time of the poor is less productive on the average than the time of the medical staff. Thus, to the extent that there is a tradeoff between the waiting time of the poor patient and the idle time of staff, economic efficiency dictates that the former should wait. Yet society may be willing to sacrifice economic efficiency in delivery of health care services in order to obtain a greater equity in the delivery of these services.[8] Selecting a single access measure, such as utilization, potentially simplifies the task of reaching policy conclusions, but we find the qualitative features too important to dismiss.

Political decisions are generally made in response to various forms of constituent pressure. Evidence of widespread constituent dissatisfaction or concern often elicits political responses and ultimately affects legislative and administrative decisions. In this regard, it is useful to examine attitudinal indices relating to *individuals' satisfaction with the medical care they now personally receive,* a fourth type of access measure.

Although access concepts may be applied to any and all areas of the health care system, our study deals almost exclusively with access to physicians' services. The physician occupies a preeminent position in the health care system and is the source of referrals to other parts of the system; hence knowledge about access to physicians reveals valuable information about patient access problems in general.

Relationship of Inflation-Recession to Access

As already noted, compared to the 1960s, the performance of the U.S. economy throughout the 1970s has been poor in terms of overall economic growth, unemployment, and inflation. Moreover, economists and policymakers are seriously reassessing the notion of a tradeoff between unemployment and inflation since the United States and other countries have recently experienced so much of both. Even if one accepts the notion of a tradeoff, the terms of trade between unemployment and inflation appear to have worsened during the 1970s. Although the performance of the economy, especially gauged in terms of inflation and unemployment, has left something to be desired throughout this decade, 1974 and 1975 were particularly bad years. For this reason, and because special surveys of access were conducted then, these years receive special emphasis in this study.

There are several accounts of the causes of the recent inflation-recession and discussion of these is beyond the scope of the present study.[9] However, it is essential to understand the consequences of inflation-recession, especially those related to medical care use. There is a surprising dearth of empirical evidence on consequences of *any* inflation and/or recession, including the most recent one.

For this reason, one must rely on inferences from economic theory to a considerable degree. The fact that recession and inflation have coexisted during the 1970s, of course, makes matters much more complex.

Effects of Inflation

Important effects of inflation may be seen in terms of the aggregate output of goods and services and the distribution of those goods and services among the members of society. Inflation causes a redistribution against families with fixed incomes. It is often asserted that families on fixed incomes, including the aged and welfare families, suffer disproportionately during recession. In fact, whether real transfer payments rise or fall depends in large part on political responses to inflation. Governments may, and very often do, take actions to preserve the real value of transfer payments.

The picture for the elderly during the first half of the 1970s is mixed. Table 1-1, which presents real transfer payments data by transfer program for the years 1970-1976, indicates that real Social Security payments (OASDHI) actually rose during 1974-1975 and continued to rise in 1976 after overall economic conditions improved. Recipients of Old Age Assistance-SSI fared less well as real payments per recipient declined substantially over the 1970-1976 period. Data on private pension plan disbursements per recipient, available from the Department of Commerce, show that real private pension payments fell in 1974.[10]

Although there are exceptions, as seen in table 1-1, real transfer payments to the nonelderly poor rose in 1974, but fell in 1975; yet real payments in general remained at a higher level than in the early 1970s. AFDC recipients, who maintained their position in 1975, relative to 1974, fared somewhat better than persons in the other assistance programs, General Assistance, Aid to the Blind-SSI, and Aid to the Disabled-SSI.

Medicaid payments per recipient remained fairly constant in real terms, using either the Consumer Price Index (per recipient (1)) or the Medical Care Price Index deflators (per recipient (3)). Combining the joint effects of increased Medicaid enrollments and a constant (real) payment per recipient, the share of the total expenditures on health care services financed by Medicaid rose during 1974-1975.[11]

These figures give the good news. They reveal real income of persons receiving transfer payments on a continuing basis, but do not account for income losses associated with early retirement, job loss, and/or "discouraged worker effects."[12] Even if transfer payment recipients did not in many instances fare worse in 1974-1975 than previously, persons who became recipients as a result of deteriorating economic conditions probably were adversely affected.

Table 1-1
Real Transfer Payments, 1970–1976

	1970	1971	1972	1973	1974	1975	1976
Consumer Price Index	100.0	104.3	107.7	114.4	127.7	138.6	146.6
Medical Care Price Index	100.0	106.4	110.0	114.1	124.8	139.8	153.2
Physician Fee Index	100.0	106.9	110.2	113.8	124.3	139.5	155.3
Program							
			Mean monthly payments (1970 dollars)[a]				
Aid to Dependent Children							
per family	190	183	178	170	172	166	161
per recipient	50	50	50	50	52	52	51
General Assistance							
per case	112	107	107	107	110	104	105
Old-Age Assistance-SSI[b]	78	75	74	66	72	66	64
Aid to the Blind-SSI[b]	104	102	105	98	111	106	104
Aid for the Disabled-SSI[b]	98	98	98	96	112	102	100
OASDHI (Social Security)	117	126	123	144	146	148	153
Medicaid payments							
per recipient[a]	80	86	84	94	90	96	101
per recipient[c]	80	85	82	95	92	95	97

Sources: U.S. Department of Commerce, *Statistical Abstract of the United States, 1976* and *Statistical Abstract of the United States, 1977,* Washington: Government Printing Office; Jules H. Berman, "Medicaid Problems," *Washington Social Legislation Bulletin 25* (July 11, 1977): 49–52; U.S. Department of Health, Education, and Welfare, Social Security Administration, *Social Security Bulletin,* Vol. *41* (5) May 1978.

[a] All items except Medicaid payments per recipient are deflated by the Consumer Price Index, 1970 = 100.

[b] SSI replaced Old-Age Assistance, Aid to the Blind, and Aid for the Disabled programs in 1974.

[c] Deflated by the Medical Care Price Index (1970 = 100).

If prices of goods and services comprising the marketbaskets of elder and poor families rose more than the average, calculations in table 1-1, which are based on price indexes for the economy as a whole, would overstate real transfer payments in 1974-1975. However, using Bureau of Labor Statistics data on cost-of-living for lower, intermediate, higher budget families, and for retired couples, we have been unable to discern any meaningful differences among these groups in the growth of cost-of-living.

Second, inflation redistributes wealth from creditors to debtors. The household sector in the aggregate is the major creditor and therefore stands to lose the most from inflation. The major debtors are governments at all levels. Knowledge that the household sector is the major creditor and thereby loses from inflation does not by itself reveal the presence of adverse distributional effects within the household sector. To examine these, one must distinguish between unanticipated as opposed to anticipated inflation and between monetary and variable price assets.

If inflation is anticipated, the creditor can demand an inflation premium in advance. For example, suppose that creditors on average anticipate a 5 percent inflation rate. Then if the market return on an asset with a certain degree of risk is 5 percent, the creditor will demand a nominal return of 10 percent, 5 percent to cover price increases. If the 5 percent inflation is in fact realized, no redistribution between creditors and debtors occurs. But suppose the inflation rate rises to 10 percent, and the terms between the creditor and debtor are fixed, debtors gain and creditors lose. Certainly many creditors during recent years, both within and without the household sector, found themselves at a disadvantage since the inflation was not generally anticipated and hence was not reflected in credit agreements.

Net worth statements per se do not reveal these wealth transfers since variable price assets, including real property and durable good assets such as automobiles, appreciate in value during inflation, sometimes to greater extent than the Consumer Price Index itself. Monetary assets, including currency and bonds, do not appreciate.

Bach measured redistributional effects on the creditor-debtor account by family income and age of household head.[13] He defined a "leverage ratio," variable price assets over total assets minus debts. Families with large amounts of variable price assets are less vulnerable to unanticipated inflation; those with monetary assets are more vulnerable. Thus, low values of the leverage ratio signify vulnerability to inflation.

Bach's calculations are reproduced in table 1--2. The data correspond to 1968-1969, but there is no reason to believe that the asset-debt composition of households has changed markedly during the 1970s. The author cautioned that wealthy families' holdings of both monetary assets fixed in dollar terms and common stocks, which are variable, are seriously understated, but it is not clear what the net impact on the leverage ratio would be. The top half of the table

Table 1-2
Assets and Debts of Households, Early 1969

	Percent of All Households	Total Assets (Billions of Dollars)	Percent of Total Assets			Leverage Ratio
			Monetary Assets	Variable Price Assets	Debts	
By 1968 money income before taxes						
Under $3,000	17	92	20	80	8	0.87
3,000–4,999	14	119	20	80	15	0.94
5,000–9,999	33	350	18	82	23	1.05
10,000–14,999	24	420	14	86	29	1.22
15,000–24,999	9	359	12	88	21	1.11
25,000–49,999	2	177	14	86	18	1.05
50,000 and over	0.4	105	18	82	10	0.91
By age of head of household						
18–24	10	27	14	86	49	1.68
25–34	21	189	8	92	48	1.75
35–44	18	335	9	91	37	1.44
45–54	17	366	13	87	22	1.12
55–64	15	301	21	79	9	0.87
65 and over	19	404	23	77	3	0.80

Source: George L. Bach, "Inflation: Who Gains and Who Loses?" *Challenge* (July–August 1974):53. Reprinted with permission.

clearly implies that the very poor and very rich are most vulnerable to inflation. Both groups have leverage ratios under 1.0. The poor have few debts because, inter alia, they are poor credit risks. The very rich by contrast tend to hold large quantities of bonds. By contrast, the middle classes hold a large part of their asset portfolio in variable price assets and have higher debts in relation to wealth.

The leverage ratio declines monotonically with the household head's age with one exception. Young families borrow for purposes of buying houses, automobiles, schooling, and the like. The elderly have few debts, and monetary assets are important components of their portfolios. From this vantage point, the young and the elderly households are worse off as a consequence of inflation.

These are the potential consequences of inflation on aggregate demand and hence on the level of currently produced goods and services (Gross National Product). The aggregate effects are attributed to a change in the rate of inflation consumers anticipate. The expected rate of future inflation probably has risen as a result of the marked rise in prices experienced during the mid- and late 1970s.

Using microeconomic theory as a guide, economists have traditionally reasoned that an expected rise in prices results in a shift of planned (future) consumption to the present. This backward shift is said to occur for two reasons. First, until nominal interest rates adjust, the higher anticipated inflation rate lowers the real rate of interest. Given a lower incentive to save, households shift from current savings (for purposes of future consumption) to current consumption. Second, households expect such variable price assets as tangible property to appreciate in value, and therefore transfer their assets from various forms of fixed price to forms of tangible property, like consumer durables. In contrast to consumer nondurables and services, durables can be stored for use and/or resale at a later date. Thus, to the extent that inflation boosts consumption, there are conceptual reasons for predicting that it has the greatest impact on durables. In economic jargon, these are *intertemporal substitution effects.*

In fact, predictions from theory have often conflicted with the empirical evidence, and recent experience with inflation (for example, 1974-1975) is no exception in this regard. Both aggregate demand in general and demand for consumer durables in particular have tended to decline during inflationary periods. Furthermore, the traditional view runs counter to the empirical fact that consumers save more and in more liquid forms in response to previously unanticipated inflation.[14] These observations have led some economists to place increasing emphasis on mechanisms to explain the observed phenomena. This group of economists does not deny the existence of the above intertemporal substitution effects, but they suggest that the intertemporal substitution effects are dominated by forces operating in the opposite direction.

High rates of inflation greatly increase consumer uncertainty and the information costs associated with various market decisions. Even though they stand to lose by keeping assets in liquid forms (cash, savings accounts, short term bonds and so on), they gain flexibility in this way during the time they evaluate the alternatives. As Okun stated:

> Prolonged and intense inflation upsets many habits of economic life, confronting consumers with price increases and price dispersions that send them shopping; making them doubt their ability to maintain their living standards; and downgrade the value of their career jobs and long-term savings; and forcing them to compile more information and to try to predict the future—costly and risky activities that they are poorly qualified to execute and bound to view with anxiety.[15]

In fact, this nonquantifiable cost may be one of the worst consequences of the recent inflation. Consumers have been forced to hedge their bets, especially those in lower income brackets who cannot "afford" to make a mistake. As Juster and Wachtel noted, even if the consumer thought that the probability that his real income would rise with inflation equalled the probability of it falling, he may, as a risk-averter, hedge to avoid the consequences of a decline.[16] If the consumer acts as if he will be poorer in the future, he is likely to spend less in the present. Both anticipated and actual income losses are responsible for negative *income effects* on current spending. Income effects offset intertemporal substitution effects.

Given the above consequences of inflation in general and the most recent inflation in particular, what are the implications for medical care utilization? In 1974, referring to the high inflation rate and, to a lesser degree, rising unemployment, Karen Davis wrote:

> All Americans share in the burdens imposed by rising medical care prices. Unfortunately, however, this burden falls more heavily on those who can least afford it—low-income families and the elderly who devote a larger share of their limited incomes to health care services. Unlike higher income families, those at the low end of the income scale have few options for mitigating the impact of inflation. They find it impossible to substitute lower cost services for more expensive kinds of health care since they already seek out the lowest cost forms of health care available. Many low-income families will be forced to postpone medical care, particularly preventive care services, and thus may expect greater health problems in the future. At the same time that access to medical care services is curtailed, rising costs of essential items such as food and heating and the stresses of unemployment may well undermine the health of many.
>
> Government programs are not currently offsetting these adverse pressures. Instead lower income families and the elderly are finding reduced assistance from outside sources. The real value of public medical care programs which attempt to provide special assistance to the poor—such as the neighborhood health center program—have declined in recent years as budgetary outlays have failed to keep pace with the cost of

services. Even the Medicaid program, which has experienced rapid
increases in expenditures, now provides fewer real services per recipient
than it did in the early years of its operation. Despite Medicare, the
elderly, too, have been hard hit by inflation and now pay more for
medical care than before Medicare's initiation in 1966.[17]

At the time, Davis did not have access to data on the 1974–1975 inflation.
More recent evidence, taken in conjunction with findings from this study, support some of Davis' contentions. Although it is true that the disadvantaged have
fewer options for mitigating the effects of inflation in general, it is very risky to
make judgments about the impact of inflation on the poor on conceptual
grounds. As it turned out, real transfer payments did not decline in many of the
programs examined. Among such programs is Medicaid, which according to our
calculations maintained its purchasing power. Although out-of-pocket payments
rose under Medicare, Social Security benefits actually rose in real terms, a factor
that must be also considered in evaluating inflation's effect on the elderly. This
is not to say there is reason for complacency in this regard since some programs
offered lower real payments in the mid-1970s. Moreover, one may infer (with
some reservations) from pre-1970 data presented above that the real net asset
position of the poor and the elderly deteriorated as a direct consequence of
recent inflation, both in absolute terms and relative to other population groups.
The uncertainty generated by inflation may have had its greatest impact on the
poor, and this burden of inflation may be quite substantial.

Even a brief examination of the literature on inflation and its consequences
reveals that there is a surprising lack of empirical evidence on the subject.
Certainly the distributional effects are complex; a particular group may lose in
some respects, and, like the elderly, gain in others.

Current knowledge about the effect of inflation on consumption is quite
rudimentary. In fact, there is disagreement about inflationary impacts on such
broad commodity groups as consumer durables and nondurables and services,
much less a single commodity such as health care. There are no published
studies directly linking inflation to any of the access dimensions delineated in
the previous section.

Effects of Unemployment

The rise in unemployment followed the rapid rise in inflation of 1974, rose to a
peak in 1975, and since then has remained at levels quite high by historical
standards. In fact, the above "normal" unemployment rates of late 1974 and
subsequent years reflect government attempts to temper the inflation rate. It is
often alleged that recession has the greatest impact on the poor and near-poor
below age 65, on teenagers, and on minorities. Moreover, many assert that these

groups suffer much more from the effects of recession than from inflation. Even though there is often good reason to dispute conventional wisdom, in this instance, as reflected in table 1–3, it appears to be a target. What is unique about the performance in 1974–1975 and subsequent years is that high rates of unemployment and inflation have persisted concurrently.

Unemployment rates understate the effects of recession since many persons temporarily withdraw from the labor force and therefore are not counted among the employed. Furthermore, unemployment rates do not reflect recession-induced underemployment. Table 1–4 presents information on labor force participation rates and reasons for nonparticipation for the same period. Overall, nonparticipation rates rose for males and fell for females. The rising participation rate for females reflects a secular trend and may, of course, have risen even more rapidly in a more robust economy. Furthermore, some wives may have decided to seek work after their husbands lost their jobs. Reasons for nonparticipation are also revealing. The proportions of persons citing "ill health, disability," "retirement, old age," and "think cannot get job" rose substantially in the recession years, 1974–1975. Although the third reason is fully attributable to recession, the other two at least partly reflect improved disability coverage and increased real Social Security benefits. These are important consequences of recession that have particular relevance to our study.

First, recession causes substantial losses in real income due to unemployment and underemployment. More affluent households often experience losses in wealth as the value of their variable price assets, in particular, common stock, falls. Frequently, such losses are only paper losses, and for this reason, among others, there is considerably greater concern among policymakers about unemployment.

Table 1–3
Unemployment Trends, 1970–1976

Unemployment Rate	1970	1971	1972	1973	1974	1975	1976
All workers	4.9	5.9	5.6	5.9	5.6	8.5	7.7
Men, 20 years and over	3.5	4.4	4.0	3.2	3.8	6.7	5.9
Women, 20 years and over	4.8	5.7	5.4	4.8	5.5	8.0	7.4
Household heads	2.9	3.6	3.3	2.9	3.3	5.8	5.1
Teenagers (ages 16 to 19)	15.3	16.9	16.2	14.5	16.0	19.9	19.0
Ratio, Negro and other to white unemployment	1.8	1.8	2.0	2.1	2.0	1.8	1.9
Average duration of unemployment (weeks)	8.8	11.4	12.1	10.1	9.7	14.1	15.8

Source: U.S. Bureau of Labor Statistics, *Handbook of Labor Statistics,* Washington: U.S. Government Printing Office, April 1976.

Table 1-4
Nonparticipation in the Labor Force, by Sex, 1970-1976

Nonparticipants by Reason of Status (in Thousands, Index 1970 = 100)	1970	1971	1972	1973	1974	1975	1976
Total	100.0	102.6	104.6	105.4	106.1	108.1	108.9
In school	100.0	106.9	105.3	103.1	100.9	108.5	109.8
Ill health, disability	100.0	106.3	113.5	119.1	124.9	125.3	123.0
Home responsibilities	100.0	100.5	101.2	100.3	99.7	98.1	96.6
Retirement, old age	100.0	104.1	113.1	121.1	124.7	132.7	145.3
Think cannot get job	100.0	121.3	106.0	106.4	107.5	169.6	142.6
All other reasons	100.0	103.7	108.0	116.1	124.1	123.0	142.3
Males	100.0	104.9	108.6	111.3	114.1	120.8	125.1
In school	100.0	107.2	105.8	104.0	99.5	108.5	108.6
Ill health, disability	100.0	106.0	112.0	118.7	125.5	126.6	127.3
Home responsibilities	100.0	109.0	96.8	102.3	107.2	99.1	110.4
Retirement, old age	100.0	103.6	109.3	113.6	117.5	123.2	130.7
Think cannot get job	100.0	107.6	108.6	101.8	102.7	162.4	145.2
All other reasons	100.0	101.5	110.0	112.5	122.7	130.4	141.0
Percent *not* in labor force	19.4	20.0	20.3	20.5	20.6	21.5	21.9
Females	100.0	101.8	103.4	103.6	103.6	104.0	103.8
In school	100.0	106.4	104.7	102.1	102.2	108.4	111.1
Ill health, disability	100.0	106.5	115.2	119.5	124.3	124.0	118.5
Home responsibilities	100.0	100.3	101.2	100.3	99.6	98.0	96.5
Retirement, old age	100.0	107.4	140.7	100.3	180.0	202.4	253.2
Think cannot get job	100.0	128.5	126.1	108.9	110.1	173.1	141.5
All other reasons	100.0	105.7	106.2	119.8	125.4	129.2	143.5
Percent *not* in labor force	56.6	56.6	56.1	55.3	54.3	53.6	52.3

Source: U.S. Bureau of Labor Statistics, *Handbook of Labor Statistics*, Washington: U.S. Government Printing Office, 1976; U.S. Department of Commerce, *Statistical Abstract of the United States, 1977*, Washington: U.S. Government Printing Office, 1977.

For analytical purposes, it is useful to divide real observed income into permanent and transitory components. Permanent income is a flow from various assets in the family's portfolio, both the human and physical capital it possesses. Families base their long-run consumption decisions on this type of income. Transitory income represents unanticipated income for a given period; it is positive in "good" years, say if a person works an unusual amount of overtime, and negative in "bad" ones, for example when the person is temporarily unemployed. Short-term unemployment is not likely to affect an individual's evaluation of his long-run financial position. If it does, there is a transitory income loss, but permanent income is virtually unaffected. If unemployment persists, the jobless individual may reassess his long-run chances, and permanent income would fall as a result.

The distinction between permanent and transitory income is important for what it implies about consumption decisions. Darby and others have shown that transitory income is principally spent to build up inventories of durable goods and cash balances.[18] In good times, durable good purchases and household cash balances rise; in recessions, decreases in these items provide a temporary cushion. By contrast, consumption of nondurable goods, food, clothing, services, and the like, are reasonably independent of transitory income, but are dependent on permanent income. Hence, as bad times persist, these items too will be affected, but not in the very short run. Services are partial substitutes for durable goods. For instance, consumers may decide to repair their automobiles rather than buy new ones during adverse times. The literature implies that certain elective health care procedures would be postponed during brief economic downturns, for instance, orthodontia, eye care and eyeglasses, and cosmetic surgery. On the other hand, families may attempt to maintain past levels of consumption of many types of health care services over the short term. The increased probability of job loss may be responsible for the same types of anticipatory responses as in times of inflation. Employed persons, fearing unemployment, may act as if they are currently experiencing a loss in transitory income. Unfortunately, there is no empirical evidence concerning the type of behavior in question.

Second, a decrease in job availability causes nonmarket and unemployed time to increase. By nonmarket time, we mean time devoted to household, self-improvement activities, and leisure. Included in nonmarket time would be increases in time spent not working because of a shortened workweek. Unemployed time refers to time the unemployed spend in job search. This effect is pertinent to our study because the value individuals place on their time is a determinant of medical care utilization as well as some of the process dimensions of access, such as waiting time spent in the physician's office.

Until the 1970s, calculations of the welfare cost of unemployment implicitly assumed that the value of nonmarket and unemployed time to the individual and his family was zero.[19] Output losses associated with reductions in employment were assumed to represent the full "cost of recession." The basic deficiency of this approach is its failure to impute a positive value to activities other than those directly associated with work in the marketplace. More realistically, a fall in work hours during a recession is offset by an equal rise in the hours devoted to other activities. Since these hours are generally productive of individual and family well-being as well, they partially offset the loss in employment-related output. To see these interrelationships, assume that the "representative" adult family member has two alternatives, work in the market and work at home. The concept of work at home means that the family member can spend his time at home, or more generally outside the market producing commodities of ultimate satisfaction to his family and himself, for instance, helping children with homework or taking them on outings, home repairs, consuming health care services that presumably contribute to good health. In this sense, the home is a little factory producing final commodities demanded by the household, such as good reading skills, housing services, and good health. As defined, "work at home" includes leisure.

As in a market context, the demand for the time of the family member is derived from the demand for the final commodities consumed by family members. The value of a person's time in household production falls as he works longer hours, certainly as plausible an assumption in the context of the household as it is in the context of the market. A person who spends 100 hours a week at home (disregarding sleep time) will tend to have less valuable uses for his time at the margin that one who spends ten hours there.

Figure 1-1 shows the derived demand for home time (D) and the supply of labor (S) schedules for the family member. The derived demand schedule relates the person's "shadow wage" to the number of hours worked at home, or equivalently, in nonmarket pursuits. The shadow wage reflects the value of the additional commodities that would be produced if the person worked another hour at home. This wage will be high if the commodity is highly valued and/or if the person is productive at the margin in producing this commodity. This schedule falls as hours at home rise because marginal productivity falls.

The supply of labor schedule that reflects the amount the individual is willing to work as a function of market wages offered is the mirror image of D At a small number of work hours, a low market wage is demanded because the individual's time is less valuable in nonmarket pursuits. High wages are required by the individual for long work hours because long work hours necessarily mean short home hours and a marginal product in nonmarket activities.

At a market wage of W_1, the person will work HW_1 hours in the market and spend the remainder of his allocatable hours, HH_1, in nonmarket pursuits. Given this time allocation, at the margin, he produces W_1 worth of output per hour for his employer and W_1 per hour worth of commodities at home, his shadow wage. For employed persons, according to the model, the market wage and the shadow wage are equal. If for some reason, the latter exceeded the former, the individual would reduce his work hours (assuming he can do so freely) until equality was restored.

If the market wage fell to W_2 because of a recession, and the demand curve remained stable—an assumption to be relaxed below, the individual would allo-

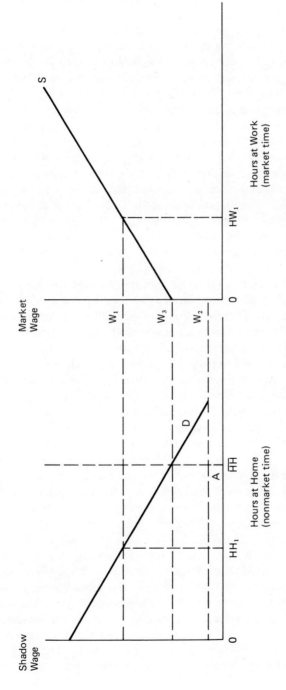

Figure 1-1. Demand for Home Time and the Supply of Labor

cate $\overline{HH}$ hours to nonmarket pursuits, where $\overline{HH}$ is the maximum number of hours available to all uses combined. Then, no time would be spent in the market. The decline in the market wage means the value of nonmarket time, or equivalently the shadow wage, has fallen from W_1 to W_3, and the market wage no longer measure the shadow wage; the shadow wage (W_3) exceeds the market wage (W_2). In nontechnical terms, it does not pay to work. While applicable to recessions, the model actually encompasses nonparticipation in the labor force for many reasons. As a general matter, a person will not participate in the labor force if his shadow wage, reflecting marginal productivity in nonmarket activity, exceeds the wage he is offered in the marketplace at zero work hours. Since S is the mirror image of D over the feasible range of hours, zero to $\overline{HH}$, an estimate of the D schedule and shadow wages, conditional on assumed values of work hours, may be obtained from an estimated labor supply schedule; this schedule may be estimated using regression analysis. Once S and D schedules have been obtained, one may estimate the shadow wage at zero work hours (W_3 in figure 1-1). We shall employ this methodology in two of the later chapters in order to estimate the shadow wage of the nonemployed in general and the unemployed in particular (assuming job search is negligible).

For purposes of exposition, we have thus far assumed that the D schedule itself is fixed. It can be demonstrated, however, that a decrease in household income, as frequently occurs in a recession, shifts the derived demand from home labor schedule D downward as the family consumption falls. Intuitively, if a trip to Florida is postponed, the adult family member's time is not needed to drive the car; or if visits to the physician are postponed, less of his or her time is needed for this type of activity as well. Thus, if the loss of employment at wage W_1 is accompanied by a sufficiently large downward shift in D (to allow an intersection of time constraint line $\overline{HH}$ and the W_2 line below A), the individual would accept a job paying W_2 after all. At issue is the sensitivity of consumption to income losses in the short run. If the family tries to maintain its former life style, the model predicts that the individual will hold out for another job with a wage of at least W_3. Whether or not he does is an empirical issue.

A third consequence of recession follows from the second and is the reason that the shadow wage concept is pertinent to this study. Loss of employment reduces the individual's price of time in nonmarket activities. As a result, the nonemployed person is more likely to purchase goods and services which require higher amounts of his own time to use. Increasingly, it is recognized that the price of goods or services is not exclusively the out-of-pocket money price. For example, the total price of a visit to a physician's office consists of the fee minus the amount paid by insurance, out-of-pocket payments for carfare and the direct expenditures, *and* the value of the total time the patient spends in obtaining care. The time cost is equal to the product of the amount of time spent and the shadow wage. If the shadow wage falls as a result of recession, the total time price declines as well. Given a negative demand schedule for office visits, the fall in the total price will result in an increased demand for visits, holding all other factors constant. Furthermore, since time has a lower value, the patient may choose more time-intensive methods of health services consumption, for example, take the bus rather than a taxi, choose providers requiring longer patient waits but at the same time charging a lower out-of-pocket price. The patient may, for example, select a hospital outpatient clinic rather than a private practitioner.

It is entirely possible that because of the time factor, job loss leads to greater use of physicians' services because the person now "has the time." The decline in income associated with loss of employment is however one of the forces operating to decrease utilization. Which of these opposing forces dominates cannot be determined a priori; empirical evidence concerning the effects of unemployment is needed to settle this issue.

A fourth consequence of recession involves the loss of private health insurance coverage. Lee estimated that during the 1974–1975 recession between 875,000 and 1,071,000 households lost health insurance at any one time as a result of job loss of the household head.[20] Only a small proportion (10 to 14 percent) of workers losing group coverage substituted individual nongroup for group coverage. To a limited extent, Medicaid and related sources of coverage filled the gap. Not surprisingly, the pattern of health insurance losses in 1974–1975 were greatest for young, nonwhite, and female workers, groups that generally suffered the most from recession. Since the shift from private to public health insurance coverage was an important consequence of the recession, the role of both private and public insurance as access determinants is emphasized in this study.

Fifth, the work of Brenner established a link between unemployment and health status, as measured by a number of types of mortality and mental hospital admissions.[21] Brenner also attempted to gauge the impacts of inflation and per capita income on health status; the results in the case of inflation were suggestive of an impact, but the impact was not as consistently strong as in the case of unemployment. The results for per capita income were the least reliable of the three. In fact, while per capita income demonstrated an overall negative effect on mortality, for mortality from cardiovascular diseases, income had the opposite effect. Positive associations between mortality and personal income have been reported in other studies.[22]

Summary and Conclusions

This chapter has provided a brief definition of access to health care services, has discussed trends in inflation and recession during the 1970s, as well as the rather subtle impacts adverse economic conditions have on household decision-making in general and utilization of health care services in particular. Because of many offsetting influences, inferences about household responses to adverse conditions, based on economic theory, or for that matter, the theory of any other discipline, will not take one very far. Furthermore, generalizations about who loses in inflation are difficult to make, since no two inflationary periods are exactly alike, and governments' decisions in the area of transfer payment policy are likely to differ, depending on the country's political climate. In the final analysis, the question of who gains and who loses in particular inflations is an empirical one. Generalizations about recessions are somewhat easier since the economically disadvantaged are frequently the "first fired and last hired." But, nevertheless, the importance of empirical research on specific recessions *and* their effects cannot be overemphasized.[23]

Notes

1. Anne R. Somers, *Health Care in Transition: Directions for the Future,* Chicago: Hospital Research and EducationalTrust, 1971, p. 23.

2. Ronald Andersen, Joanna Lion, and Odin Anderson, *Two Decades of Health Services: Social Survey Trends in Use and Expenditure,* Cambridge, Massachusetts: Ballinger Publishing Company, 1976; The Robert Wood Johnson Foundation, *Special Report on Access—America's Health Care System: A Comprehensive Portrait,* Princeton, New Jersey (forthcoming). David E. Rogers and Robert J. Blendon, "The Changing American Health Scene: Sometimes Things Get Better," *Journal of the American Medical Association,* 237 (April 18, 1977):1710-1714.

3. See Thomas Juster and Paul Wachtel, "Anticipatory and Objective Models of Durable Goods Demand," *Brookings Papers on Economic Activity* 1 (1975):71-121; Susan Burch and Diane Werneke, "The Stock of Consumer Durables, Inflation, and Personal Savings Decisions," *Review of Economics and Statistics* 59 (1975):141-54; William L. Springer, "Consumer Spending and the Rate of Inflation," *Review of Economics and Statistics* 59 (August 1977):299-306.

4. Ronald Andersen, Joanna Kravits, and Odin Anderson, *Equity in Health Services: Empirical Analyses in Social Policy,* Cambridge, Massachusetts: Ballinger Publishing Co., 1975, p. 10. Reprinted with permission.

5. A useful review of cultural and social factors underlying illness and illness behavior is David Mechanic, *Public Expectation and Health Care; Essays on the Changing Organization of Health Services,* New York: Wiley-Interscience, 1972.

6. Stephen Cole and Robert LeJeune assess the use of illness as a means of coping with failure in their article "Illness and Legitimization of Failure," *American Sociological Review* 37 (June 1972):347-356.

7. David Salkever, "Economic Class and Differential Access to Care: Comparisons Among Health Care Systems," *International Journal of Health Services* 5 (Summer 1975):373-395.

8. In brief, economic efficiency means securing the maximum amount of goods and services from a fixed amount of scarce resources—land, raw materials, capital, and labor. The relationship between waiting time and economic efficiency is developed in Frank Sloan and John Lorant, "The Role of Waiting Time: Evidence from Physicians' Practices," *Journal of Business* 50 (October): 486–507, 1977; it is discussed somewhat more indirectly in Barry Schwartz, *Queuing and Waiting: Studies in the Social Organization of Access and Delay,* Chicago: University of Chicago, 1975.

9. William Nordhaus and John Shoven, "Inflation 1973: The Year of Infamy," *Challenge* (May–June 1974):14–22.

10. U.S. Department of Commerce, *Statistical Abstract of the United States, 1977,* Washington: U.S. Government Printing Office, 1977.

11. U.S. Department of Health, Education, and Welfare, Social Security Administration, Office of Research and Statistics, "National Health Expenditure Highlights, Fiscal Year 1976," *Research and Statistics Note,* No. 27, December 22, 1976.

12. A worker is said to be discouraged if he or she stays out of the labor force because of poor job prospects. For a discussion of the discouraged workers, see William G. Bowen and T. Aldrich Finegan, *The Economics of Labor Force Participation,* Princeton, New Jersey: Princeton University Press, 1969.

13. George L. Bach, "Inflation: Who Gains and Who Loses?" *Challenge* (July–August 1974):48–55.

14. George Katona, "Change in Consumer Expectations and Their Origin," in *The Quality and Economic Significance of Anticipations Data,* Princeton, New Jersey: Princeton University Press, 1960; Juster and Wachtel, supra, note 3.

15. Arthur M. Okun, "Inflation: Its Mechanics and Welfare Costs," *Brookings Papers on Economic Activity* 2 (1975):351–401. Reprinted with permission.

16. Juster and Wachtel, *Anticipatory and Objective Models.*

17. Karen Davis, "The Impact of Inflation and Unemployment on Health Care of Low-Income Families," in Michael Zubkoff (ed.), *Health: A Victim or Cause of Inflation?* New York: Prodist, 1976, pp. 55–69. Reprinted with permission.

18. Michael R. Darby, "The Allocation of Transitory Income Among Consumers' Assets," *American Economic Review* (1972):928–941.

19. Arthur M. Okun, "Potential GNP: Its Measurement and Significance," in American Statistical Association, *Proceedings of the Business and Economics Statistics Section* (1962):98–104; "Inflation: Its Mechanics and Welfare Costs," *Brookings Papers on Economic Activity* 2 (1975):351–401.

20. James A. Lee, *Employment, Unemployment, and Health Insurance,* Cambridge, Massachusetts: Abt Books, 1979.

21. M. Harvey Brenner, *Estimating Social Costs of National Economic Policy: Implications for Mental and Physical Health and Criminal Aggression,* Washington: Joint Economic Committee of the U.S. Congress, October 26, 1976.

22. Richard Auster, Irving Levenson, and Deborah Sarachek, "The Production of Health: An Exploratory Study," *Journal of Human Resources* 4 (Fall 1969):411–436.

23. A recent article by Lester Thurow, "The Real Sources of Economic Pain," *Wall Street Journal,* July 6, 1978, p. 10, suggests that the personal income distribution in the U.S. changed imperceptibly between 1973 and 1976, despite the economic turbulence of the intervening years. Although some of the data we have presented, in transfer payments, for example, is inconsistent with this, we cannot conclude that no meaningful shifts occurred during this period. First, Thurow's income categories are broad (quintiles). Second, conditions improved in 1976 vis-a-vis 1974 and 1975. Employees' wages may have caught up with inflation by this time. Third, Thurow's data are for income classes; certain racial and age groups may have been affected even if the personal income distribution by income class remained unchanged. Thurow emphasized that inflation can have important psychological effects on families; these are not reflected in the personal income distribution figures.

2

Past Research on Access to Ambulatory Care

Analyses of Perspectives and Responses

This chapter reviews previous studies on access to ambulatory care. This review assembles results from previous studies having implications for analysis of the impact of inflation-recession on access, provides guidance for the specification of our own access regressions, and presents baseline data representing years in which economic conditions were more favorable for purposes of comparison with more recent data presented for the first time in this study. The studies are by no means homogeneous in terms of methodology or in terms of the nature of data bases analyzed.

Before turning to specific studies, we distinguish between studies that view behavior from a macro (system) perspective versus a micro (individual) perspective. We then distinguish between short-run and long-run responses to changes in variables exogenous to the health care system.

Macro Versus Micro Perspective

The economist's model of supply and demand provides a useful starting point. This is the macro or market perspective. In the simplest of models, physicians supply quantities of homogeneous units of service for specified prices, more service being offered at higher prices. On the demand side, consumers demand units of service at specified prices, less being demanded at higher prices. Equilibrium price and quantity are established at the point of intersection of the supply and demand curves. If either recession or inflation leads to reduced demand, this model clearly implies a fall in both equilibrium price and output. In the face of increases in the prices of inputs to physicians' practices, the supply curve shifts upward; equilibrium price rises and quantity, or equivalently, utilization falls. With demand curves shifting down and supply curves shifting up, as could have conceivably occurred during the mid- and late-1970s, the model predicts a decline in utilization of physicians' services in response to inflation-recession.

This supply-demand model as applied to this market is subject to a number of criticisms. The nature of one's critique depends in large part on the nature of one's inquiry. *In the present context,* this model is deficient in acknowledging qualitative aspects of physicians' services. As noted in the previous chapter, the general term "access" is not limited to utilization. Qualitative dimensions are also included. Some of these are captured in such process variables as the amount of personal attention that physicians give to patients (roughly measured by the length of visit), patient waiting time in physicians' offices, delays between the time the appointment is made and the visit. Not only are these qualitative dimensions associated with the use of services, but they command interest in their own right. Many, for example, would view the long waits the poor experience in clinics as an injustice, irrespective of the effects patient waiting might have on utilization rates.

The notion of quality, as defined by the economist, is not limited to types of treatment that produce better health. The term encompasses amenities included in access studies as process variables. Since quality in the medical sense, though important, is difficult to measure at best and is extremely elusive to characterize when one deals with the health system as a whole, we shall confine our remarks to the above kinds of amenities. To avoid confusion, we shall refer to the qualitative dimensions as amenities.

The supply-demand model can be expanded by considering physicians as selling both quantity of service (q) and amenities associated with services (A). Just as the production of q requires resources, such as physician and aide time, supplies, and equipment, the production of amenities is resource-using. If physicians are to regularly provide instantaneous service to patients, they will have to operate at excess capacity on the average. Likewise, "humane" treatment of patients is also resource-intensive, holding other factors constant. For this reason, higher levels of A will, like higher q, be offered at higher prices.

We are now in a position to expand the above model to one in which equilibrium q, A, and price (p) are determined in the marketplace. On the demand side, consumers possess demand curves in which the quantity demanded (q) depends on price, amenities offered by the physician, and exogenous factors such as patient income, insurance coverage, and medical need. The degree to which amenities determine demand varies among individuals. For example, persons with high shadow wages are particularly sensitive to office waiting time and tend to select physicians requiring comparatively short waits. Patients with complex chronic illnesses tend to be especially concerned that they receive adequate explanations about their illnesses and the course of treatment; therefore, they eschew physicians with hurried styles. Parents with small children may stress the ability to consult with physicians during nights and weekends and hence prefer physicians who respond to patient concerns in this regard. Insurance coverage in this expanded model relates to A as well as to q. Major medical insurance, the primary source of private third-party coverage for physicians' services, subsidizes q and A. This form of insurance pays the greater part of the physician's "reasonable" fee, once the deductible has been satisfied. To the extent that third-party payers consider most fees in the distribution of physicians' fees to be "reasonable," covered patients can purchase high amenity services and have most of the difference in price between a high and a low amenity physician paid by the third party. Therefore, patients with major medical coverage, as well as high income patients, should be likely to favor physicians offering a variety of amenities. Community demand curves, the sum of individual demand curves, reflect characteristics of individuals in the community. Referring to the New York City area, demand curves in Scarsdale are undoubtedly quite different from Bedford-Stuyvesant, and the inter-community variation in equilibrium values of q, A and p are partially determined by these differences.

On the supply side, physicians are faced with decisions about how much q and A to supply. The production of q and A is competitive in the sense that both q and A draw on a common set of resources. Inputs devoted to one use cannot be allocated to another. For example, consider a physician who currently spends five minutes asking questions about the patient's medical history. To expand this function, that is, to ask additional questions of patients, the physician must (a) expand his workday, (b) see fewer patients, and/or (c) raise practice "productivity." Assuming the practice is already efficient, he can further expand his work hours or see fewer patients. If he is already working long hours, he is likely to select the latter alternative. Quite similar scenarios would apply to giving free advice over the telephone to existing patients, to reducing patient waiting time, which in turn leads to greater physician and staff waiting time, and to other amenities. Since the prices of practice inputs, including physician time, differ among communities *and* over time, the amounts of q and A forthcoming at any fee also vary.

The analytics of this model, when *both* supply and demand sides are combined are rather complex and are beyond the scope of this study.[1] A few general remarks will help in understanding the potential, limitations, and implications of our model. In particular, consider the following cases.

First, assume that expanded medical school enrollments eventually raise the physician-population ratio, which implies less demand for visits per physician in a given community. As q *and* the physician's workday fall, the physician's shadow wage falls, making it less expensive at the margin for him to offer amenities. At a lower wage, a moment of the physician's idle time is less costly, and the motive to save physician time by having patients wait is lessened; the mean length of visit may be expanded at a lower cost. So one observes shorter queues of all types, lengthier discussions between patients and physicians, and so on. These qualitative changes in turn have a positive feedback on visit demand (demand for q). Although utilization (q) may be in the final analysis still lower than before the physician-population ratio rose, amenities will be higher.

Second, say that a generous form of national health insurance were instituted that subsidized both q and A. Now patients would desire to visit physicians more frequently and at the same time demand more "conveniences" at the time services were received. In the short run, patients cannot have both unless additional resources are attracted from other sectors. To accomplish this may require substantial price increases. If patients are more intent on purchasing additional visits, amenity levels may fall at the same time price rises. The same scenario may be run in reverse when a recession results in substantial losses in private health insurance coverage. List prices may not fall, but bad debts and reduced-fee service may increase.[2]

As noted in chapter 1, cyclical unemployment accounts for reduced shadow wages *and* transitory income losses. Since the total price of a visit to a physician consists of the time price as well as an out-of-pocket money price, the total price falls, holding other factors constant, when the shadow wage falls. This fall in price should stimulate the demand for visits in communities with high unemployment and possibly increase observed office waiting times, since patients on the average find waits less costly. At the same time, transitory income losses would decrease the demand for q and amenities of all types. Which of the two offsetting effects dominates, the time price or the transitory income loss effect, is an empirical issue.

Inflation also has offsetting impacts on patient demand for visits and amenities. According to the intertemporal substitution effect, explained in chapter 1, demand would increase in the current period. This force, however, may be offset by an uncertainty-income effect which tends to depress current consumption.

A large number of studies focus on *either* the demand (consumer) or the supply (physician) sides of the market. For lack of a better term, we refer to these as "micro studies." Ideally, a study of one side of the market should be conducted at the lowest possible level of aggregation, in this context, the consumer or the physician. More aggregated observational units such as cities, states, and/or countries, are appropriate in macro or, equivalently, market-oriented studies. There are also important theoretical differences. Most important, when one side of the market is analyzed in isolation from the other, the product price is treated as exogenous (that is, determined outside the model). If amenities are included as utilization or supply determinants, they too are exogenous. By contrast, the macro studies treat both product prices and amenities as endogenous.

For purposes of this review, we shall limit the discussion of micro studies to the demand side.[3] Utilization studies, by far the most prevalent, examine the effects of fees, insurance, wages and income, educational attainment, measures of need, travel time, in a very few cases office waiting time, appointment delays on visits to physicians, and total expenditures on physicians' services. There are also a few studies that essentially examine the demand for specific amenities even though the authors often have not cast the studies in these terms. In these cases, the amenity variables themselves are the dependent variables.

Some demand models have been organized on the basis of a framework developed by Andersen.[4] Since we shall also classify explanatory variables on this basis in our work, it is worth briefly discussing elements of this scheme.

According to Andersen's model, a person's decision to seek medical care and the volume of services sought depends on the predisposition of the individual to use services (predisposing factors), the individual's ability to secure services (enabling factors), and the individual's need (need factor). Predisposing factors include patient age, ethnicity, education, ahd household head's occupation. Some of these factors, such as age, reflect need as well as tastes, but their roles as taste measures are emphasized when more direct measures of need are included, such as symptoms, disability status, and self-evaluated health status. Enabling factors include health insurance coverage, earned and nonemployment-related income, prices (both time and money), appointment delays, and proxies for physician and bed availability. The precise list, of course, depends on the nature of the dependent demand variable being analyzed. If the appointment delay is the dependent variable, it would be excluded from the list of enabling (explanatory) variables.

Micro studies have potential value for policy purposes, but it is also essential to recognize their limitations. They are useful, for instance, in assessing the impact of job loss on utilization and process variables if job loss is not too widespread. If, to continue our example, one found that unemployed persons tend to demand care from emergency rooms, one could safely assume that actual emergency room use will increase with job loss. However, if very large numbers of unemployed simultaneously sought care from such facilities, one could no longer assume that all of the demand would be accommodated at the previous price. In the long run, one would have to consider the supply response.[5] To generalize, projections based on micro demand studies assume that supply is perfectly elastic, and projections based on micro supply studies assume that demand is perfectly elastic. The macro supply-demand studies yield more reliable estimates to substantial changes in exogenous variables.

Long-Term Versus Short-Term Responses

The vast majority of econometric studies in the health care field in general and on access in particular are based on single cross-sections. Widespread use of cross-sectional data partly reflects the paucity of time-series data in this field. Cross-sectional studies permit inferences about long-term responses to changes in exogenous variables; they yield no evidence on short-run behavior or on the adjustment process from an initial response to a final equilibrium. Short-run phenomena dominate business cycles. For this reason, cross-sectional evidence is more useful for an assessment of prolonged adverse conditions than for short-lived downturns. Since the current prognosis is for sustained high unemployment and inflation for the rest of the 1970s, an assessment of long-term effects merits policy interest.

Organization of Literature Review

We divide pertinent studies into (a) physician services utilization, (b) process, and (c) satisfaction with care received. Unfortunately, there is no pertinent analytic work on the third access dimension, but some conclusions can be drawn from the descriptive evidence. This review emphasizes economic research. No attempt is made to give adequate coverage to the rich sociological and psychological literature on this subject.

Physician Services Utilization

The literature on physician services utilization and its determinants can be divided into macro descriptive studies and micro multivariate cross-sectional studies with the consumer as the observational unit.

At the national level, it is evident that visit rates have been rising over time, especially for low income groups. Rogers and Blendon, using published and unpublished data from the National Center for Health Statistics, reported that in 1975 low-income persons were seeing physicians at a rate of slightly more than six visits annually, compared with a national mean of about five.[6] Slightly over a decade earlier, not only was the gap between these two utilization rates markedly smaller, but the gap between utilization rates of high-income and low-income persons was sizable. Disaggregating further, Rogers and Blendon determined that children from low-income families in the one- to five-year age group had lower visit rates in 1976 than in 1970, although both the difference between high- and low-income visit rates narrowed. Visit rates for the elderly remained rather constant between 1970 and 1976; the poor continued to have slightly lower utilization and the gap between high- and low-income utilization widened slightly. Rising physician visit rates for the United States as a whole have also been documented by others.[7]

Since the health status of the poor, on average, tends to be relatively low, comparisons of need-adjusted utilization by income class show that inequalities persist, although there is some evidence that the gaps narrowed over the period covered by the data.[8] Need is measured in these studies on the basis of disability days and a symptoms-response ratio based on reported symptoms, weighted according to illness severity (as judged by a panel of physician consultants).

The first cross-sectional regression demand study we shall review, which is by Benham and Benham, employed a more comprehensive measure of family income than the above descriptive studies.[9] Their income measure identifies a broader range of income categories, not only high versus low income or poverty versus non-poverty. Furthermore, their income variable was constructed to measure long-term or permanent income. Two sets of equations were estimated with mean visits per year and the proportion of individuals visiting a physician as dependent variables. Permanent income and age were explanatory variables in the first set of regressions. Comparing 1963 and 1970, it is evident that permanent income had a much smaller effect on utilization in 1970 than in 1963. When symptom and disability day measures of health status were included in a second set of regressions, the effects of permanent income on use disappeared entirely in the 1970 regressions. The authors attributed the decline in the role of income to the introduction of Medicare and Medicaid. One may infer from this study that permanent income losses would not affect patient demand for physicians' services, assuming that government health insurance is available. Also, to the extent that the types of structural changes observed by Benham and Benham have occurred, analysts should be cautioned against using parameter estimates based on old data for policy purposes.[10] Benham and Benham's results do not contradict the aforementioned findings with respect to use-need. They do suggest that once one has controlled for health status, which tends to be lower in lower income families, income did not have an independent effect on demand by 1970.

Salkever assessed the relationship between need and the probability of entering the health care system for treatment.[11] He reported essentially no differences in use relative to need for adults, but children from higher level income families did have better access. Salkever's analysis was based on 1968–1969 data from Canada, England, Finland, and Poland as well as from the United States. Surprisingly, the above conclusions seem to hold for all health systems examined. In terms of structure, these systems are quite heterogeneous.

The theory establishing the role of time costs in demand analysis is now well known.[12] However, attempts to measure the role of time as a barrier to health services use are still in their infancy. Since the role of time as well as other variables such as income and insurance coverage is central to the model outlined above, this aspect will be emphasized in our review of micro demand equation models. To date, the results on the role of time as a demand determinant have been mixed.

Newhouse and Phelps assessed patient demand for physician visits, using data from a 1963 survey conducted by the University of Chicago's Center for Health Administration Studies (CHAS).[13] Newhouse and Phelps' specification was more complete than Benham and Benham's, who employed the same data base. Family income tended to have insignificant impact on demand for visits, and the associated elasticities were low. Insurance variables sometimes demonstrated a statistically significant effect on utilization, but the associated elasticities were low (0.1 or less). Newhouse and Phelps attempted to isolate the effect of time costs on visit demand, assuming that the market wage varies positively with the shadow wage. Presumably as market wages rise, time costs rise and utilization falls. Wage income elasticities, however, were found to be small and statistically insignificant.

Using data from a 1970 CHAS survey, an update of the 1963 survey, Phelps estimated demand equations with physician visits and expenditures as dependent variables. The effect of private health insurance was reported to be somewhat higher than in the work by Newhouse and Phelps (elasticities of 0.18 and 0.19 at a coinsurance rate of 25 percent); income had an insignificant effect on visit demand and a significant effect on expenditures but the associated elasticity was low (0.11). Health status measures on the whole appeared to be more important utilization determinants, at least gauged in terms of statistical significance.

The 1970 CHAS survey asked the respondent to estimate *usual* travel, office waiting time, and appointment delays with reference to his *regular* source of medical care. These questions were not asked if the respondent had no regular source. Phelps' explanatory variables for travel and waiting time were the products of the time estimates and the respondent's weekly wage. So defined, these variables measure time prices.

The same procedure was not followed for appointment delays. As Phelps noted, the appointment delay does not involve a direct cost in the same sense as travel and waiting time. Appointment delay time can generally be used for other purposes. However, if the patient is limited by his illness and cannot function in his usual manner, a delay does involve a loss of productive time, as do travel and waiting time. Some illnesses are by nature self-limiting and postponing access to the doctor may lead to a cancelled appointment. While delays are costless in the latter sense, they nevertheless may function as a utilization deterrent.

As a group, travel time, waiting time, and appointment delay variables demonstrated a small impact on the utilization of physician services in the Phelps study. At least to some extent, these poor results are attributable to inadequacies in variable measurement. We have found in our surveys that respondents often have difficulties in establishing *one* usual source of medical care; more important, it is very difficult for the respondent to give a *usual* visit or delay at a regular source. Waits and delays vary a great deal from visit to visit.

To our knowledge, the only published studies that specifically analyze the patient's choice of visit site are by Acton.[14] Both studies are based on a theory of the household in which the household maximizes utility subject to both goods and time constraints. Arguments in the utility function are medical care services and a composite good representing all other goods. Comparative static analysis based on the Acton model yields four predictions.

First, time may be expected to function as a price in studies of medical care demand. The own-time price elasticity should be negative and the cross-time price elasticity should be positive. In particular, the own-price effect implies that outpatient department visits fall when the price of such care rises. On the other hand, the cross-price effect implies that if the price of a private physician visit rises, the demand for hospital outpatient care rises.

Second, the time-price elasticity depends in part on the importance of the time price as a fraction of the total price. Holding other factors constant, as this fraction increases, the time-price elasticity increases. Thus, comparing two persons, A and B, and assuming A has a high shadow wage and B a relatively low one, the time-price elasticity should be higher, holding other factors constant, for A than for B. If B's shadow wage is currently low because he is unemployed, the model predicts that his utilization will be comparatively insensitive to the time he must travel and wait in order to obtain care. For this reason, such persons may select practice settings which tend to be patient time intensive.

Third, the effect of a change in nonearned income (from such sources as assets or welfare) on utilization of services in a particular setting is likely to vary. If consumers regard a hospital outpatient department as an "inferior" good, demand for care in this setting may be expected to rise in response to income loss. By contrast, if demand for care by office-based specialists is a "normal" good, a fall in income will lead to decreased demand for physicians in that setting. The effect of nonearned income on the demand for physicians' services, taken as a whole, is probably positive, although, as we have noted, the effect seems to be weakening over time.

Fourth, the effect of a change in a person's wage on his demand for physicians' services cannot be determined in advance. The wage effect embodies a "pure" income effect and a substitution effect. The "pure" income effect, measured by the effect of nonearned income, is positive. The substitution effect may be positive or negative, as Acton demonstrated. Its sign depends on the relative patient time intensity of physicians' services as contrasted with other goods and services. If the consumption of physicians' services is comparatively time intensive, a rise in the wage will cause a shift from physicians' services to other goods and services. Conversely, a fall in wages during a recession would stimulate demand for physicians' services. This result also applies to the patient's choice of source of care. If the consumption of clinic services requires a greater patient time input than the consumption of private physician services, a wage decrease may be expected to produce a shift from private physicians to clinics. One must, however, be careful to recognize the limitations of inferences exclusively derived from a demand study. For example, if the demand curve for private physicians' services and clinics shifted to the left and right, respectively, time costs in clinics may be expected to rise relative to those in private offices. This effect in turn would encourage some patients to return to office-based physicians.

Acton specified and estimated a simultaneous equation model, including equations for annual outpatient visits and visits to private physicians, with data from a 1965 survey of users of outpatient departments of New York City municipal hospitals.[16] Acton was more successful than Newhouse-Phelps and Phelps in isolating the effect of time costs on utilization. Outpatient clinic visits and visits to private physicians were seen to reflect travel time in part. He found that when waits at clinics exceed waits at private practitioners, the patient is more likely, holding other factors constant, to select the latter. Furthermore, his results showed that as wages rise, the patient is more likely to select a private physician. Wage and income elasticities, however, were consistently low.

A second study by Acton,[17] based on another New York City sample, investigated the roles of travel time and office waiting time on utilization of ambulatory care services. Travel and waiting time variables were based on the same questions as those in the 1970 CHAS survey, but Acton's empirical results were more definitive than Phelps', who used 1970 CHAS data. Travel time utilization elasticities reported by Acton are substantial, as high as one in absolute value. Those for waiting time are at most one-fifth as large. Since the equation specifications and the samples differ, it is virtually impossible to determine why time variables perform well in Acton's work and appear to be inconsequential in Phelps' work.[18]

With some important exceptions, empirical studies of the demand for physicians' services have been plagued by inconsistent findings and low t-values. At present the underlying theory of demand is far ahead of empirical research in the area. Since empirical research on this topic is still in its infancy, it is far too soon to attribute poor results to an inadequate theoretical foundation.

Sloan analyzed patient choice of type of physician, based on 1969 National Center for Health Statistics Health Interview Survey data merged with data from other sources.[19] Since, as argued further in chapter 5, several process variables are systematically related to provider type, a discussion of this study provides a useful transition between the present and the following sections.

In the Sloan study, the patient chooses among the following five types of physicians: general practitioner, either in a private office or in a hospital outpatient setting; specialist in either of these two settings; and hospital emergency rooms. Patients are known to wait longer in institutional settings, and experience longer appointment delays when an appointment is made.[20] It is widely believed that care is more impersonal in institutional settings as the physician tends to have overall responsibility for the care of the individual patient.[21] Furthermore, specialists have had greater amounts of training and may be perceived to offer higher quality services on the average. For these reasons, Sloan predicted that choice of provider should relate systematically to the patient's ability to pay, as measured by income and insurance coverage, that individual's shadow wage, the patient's medical condition, the relative availability of physicians in the five types of settings, and the patient's race, which may reflect a number of factors including discrimination.

The results imply that an office-based specialist tends to be chosen with a high probability by persons with high ability to pay, measured in terms of wages, family income, and private insurance coverage. When other factors are held constant, Medicaid recipients are far less likely to visit such physicians (even though it must also be said that the partial effect of Medicaid is not statistically significant at conventional levels). The availability of alternative provider types also accounted for variation in patients' choices. That is, where general practitioners are rare and hospital-based physicians relatively plentiful, the patient is more likely to select the latter. Whites are more likely, *ceteris paribus*, to eschew institutional providers. Overall, patients visiting office-based specialists stand out as a distinct group. The differences between characteristics of patients visiting office-based general practitioners and those going to institutional-based providers were found to be much smaller.

Process Variables

In contrast to analytic research on the utilization of physicians' services, most work on process variables has a macro orientation. Dependent variables in the macro studies are functions of exogenous demand and supply influences. The process studies logically fall into three categories. The first type considers short-run impacts on travel, waiting time, and appointment delays attributable to the introduction of universal health insurance. Evidence from these "before insurance-after insurance" studies suggests potential effects of an exogenous shock on the health system, although, as we shall see, one must exercise caution in applying information derived from such situations to other contexts. A second kind of study is based on cross-sectional data on individual physician practices. Such studies are "macro" in the sense that each physician is assumed to have "local" monopoly power. As a local monopolist, the physician faces a downward sloping demand curve for his services rather than a horizontal demand curve in the competitive case. While the before-after studies suggest ways in which the health system equilibrates in the short run, inferences from the studies of physicians' practices relate exclusively to long-run responses. Third, we shall review one micro study based on patient data from Washington, D.C.

Effects of Introducing Universal Insurance Coverage

A series of articles by Enterline, McDonald, and their colleagues on the effects of introducing Medicare, Canadian universal health insurance, in Quebec, provides a rich source of information on short-run responses to a "shock" to the health system.[22] Data were obtained from patients and physicians during two eight-month periods before and soon after Medicare was introduced (1969–1970 and 1971–1972).

According to these studies of patient responses, visits were unchanged in the aggregate, although the poor gained relative to the rich. Also noteworthy is their finding that the proportions of patients with specified symptoms tended to rise. Travel time and overall rates of satisfaction with care received changed very little. Since patient and physician locations are reasonably fixed in the short run, the pattern with regard to travel time is hardly surprising. Mean waiting time and appointment delays rose substantially. The access of the poor to physicians, though worse with respect to both dimensions, did not deteriorate as much as did the access of the nonpoor.

Enterline et al. reported results from the survey of physicians wherein a slight rise (4.8 percent) in the number of face-to-face contacts is apparent. Visit mix, however, changed substantially. Telephone calls and home visits fell precipitously (41.1 percent and 62.9 percent, respectively) while office visits rose substantially (32.2 percent). Physician length of visit fell slightly (4.0 percent) in the aggregate, but decreases for office and hospital visits were pronounced (15.8 percent and 15.0 percent).

The Quebec experience can be explained by a quantity-amenity model such as that described in the first section of this chapter. However, it is essential to note that physicians have been reimbursed on the basis of fixed-fee schedules rather than major medical type insurance. When prices are fixed, there are greater incentives for the growth in the number of units, possibly at the cost of quality-amenities.

As in the model, the physician may be viewed as offering q and A and facing a fixed price per unit of q.[23] Dimensions of A include office waiting time, appointment delays, length of visit, and telephone "visits" and house calls to existing patients for which there is no charge, or, in the case of home visits, a charge far below the marginal cost to the physician of providing this service. Considering the added demand pressure for q, especially from low-income groups, and the fixed-fee schedule, the system equilibrates in the short run by decreases in A. Did access improve as a result of the introduction of Medicare? The answer clearly depends on the weights one is willing to assign to the multifaceted outcomes. The multidimensional character of response cannot be emphasized enough. Certainly a single access indicator would be highly misleading in this case.[24]

Can one run the scenario in reverse to derive predictions on the impact of inflation-recession? If the only effect of adverse economic conditions were to shift the demand curve inward (and again assuming variable fees), the answer would be a "qualified yes." The reason for qualifying our response is that even such an ample change requires that one make a few plausible restrictions on the model.[25] Having made these, one can predict that q will fall and A rise in response to the demand shift. But considering that shadow wages can be expected to fall for the unemployed, and that these individuals should therefore find queues less costly, it is doubtful, at least conceptually, that *all* important dimensions of A would improve. Physicians might spend more time with each patient, but waiting time in the office might remain about the same. Certainly when one complicates matters by considering inflationary effects on the supply side, all predictions based on theory alone are off, at least with respect to A. An upward shift in the supply curve of physicians' services would, *ceteris paribus,* lower both *q* and *A*.

Because of these complexities, one cannot rely on plausible inferences from theory. The short-run effects of adverse economic conditions must be settled on the basis of empirical evidence. Nevertheless, the Quebec experience does serve to emphasize that the short-run effects of shocks to the medical care system, in either direction, may be substantial.

Cross-Sectional Analysis of Individual Physician's Practices

Sloan and Lorant performed a cross-sectional analysis of patient waiting time in private physicians' offices with the individual physician's practice as the observational unit.[26] According to their model, physicians realize efficiency gains by having patients wait, rather than waiting themselves and leaving their staffs idle. However, physicians recognize waiting time as a demand deterrent. Under a variety of assumptions of what physicians maximize, physicians will determine the mean patient wait for their practices by comparing the marginal costs and benefits from extending the wait. Patient waiting time is expected to vary geographically, reflecting supply and demand factors. The demand factors include the patient's opportunity cost of time, private and public insurance coverage, and physician-population ratios (since the individual physician is the observational unit). The supply factors include the wage rates of ancillary personnel, and the physician's shadow wage, represented in Sloan and Lorant's work by proxy variables.

They found that practices located in areas with proportionately more low-income, elderly, female, and/or black patients tend to have longer waits. Increases in the community's physician-population ratio and in major medical insurance were estimated to decrease patient waits. Judging from the negative coefficient on the private insurance variable, Sloan and Lorant reported that a shorter time in the queue is one type of amenity subsidized by insurance. This finding implies that income and insurance losses associated with high rates of unemployment may result in lengthened queues as patients are more willing to substitute their time for that of the medical staff. It is quite possible that substantial losses of insurance coverage in a community could initially lead to a reduced mean wait because of reduced demand for visits; but if the area remained depressed, the market would eventually honor consumer preferences for low-cost, low-amenity visits.

Essentially the same methodology was used by Sloan and Lorant in their study of physician length of visit.[27] In this study, the underlying model assumes that the physician recognizes that patients value attention by him and his employees. Yet increasing the amount of time spent with patients on a per-visit basis is costly. The physician determines the length of visit by balancing the marginal gain (revenue) from expanding inputs against the marginal cost of doing so. The Sloan-Lorant model explicitly considers changes in volume or visits, patient waiting time, and visit length simultaneously. Since marginal (practice) costs are assumed to rise, the model implies that physicians already offering high volume and short visits will find it costly at the margin, holding other factors constant, to expand visit length. The regression analysis in this length-of-visit study was based on a 1973 survey of physicians' practices conducted by the American Medical Association.

Sloan and Lorant found that patient income had a significantly positive impact on mean visit length although the magnitude of the response of visit length to changes in income was small. The physician-population ratio was also reported to have had a positive impact on visit length, implying that an increase in physician availability in an area increases the input of the physician and staff per visit. However, as with income, the elasticity associated with the physician-population ratio parameter was not large. In contrast to the waiting time study, major medical insurance coverage demonstrated no effect; nor was a variable measuring Medicaid coverage in the physician's area statistically significant. Variables representing physicians' credentials and patient mix generally performed in accordance with the authors' expectations.

Length of visit was viewed by Sloan and Lorant as an amenity. Others, however, have treated the inverse of length of visit (visits/input time) as a measure of productivity.[28] These latter studies considered productivity to be "good," while the length-of-visit research essentially would consider the inverse of length of visit a "bad." Eliminating waste is clearly desirable; but if improving productivity or practice throughput per unit of input actually lowers the quality of care and/or results in inhumane or brusque treatment, patients would be worse off than previously.

Appointment delays tend to exhibit a very different relationship to family income than travel time and office waiting time, both in Quebec, as seen in the studies reviewed above, and in the United States, as seen in table 2-1. While travel and waiting time are negatively related to income, there tends to be a positive association between appointment delays and income. Presumably, patients desire ready access to physicians for medical as well as psychological reasons, and it would seem reasonable to assume that this "amenity" too is a normal good. Why then has the positive relationship been observed?

Sloan and Steinwald hypothesized that at least part of the answer relates to visit mix.[29] Many of the amenities we have identified are valued by patients irrespective of the reason for their visits. For example, except for emergencies, the disutility associated with waiting in the physician's office is likely to be fairly independent of the patient's diagnosis.

By contrast, diagnosis is probably quite important in determining the value the patient places on receiving an early appointment. A short delay may be seen as important for even such minor acute illnesses as the common cold or the

Table 2-1

Mean Travel, Waiting, and Appointment Delay Times, by Family Income
and Age, United States

Age-Family Income	Travel Time (Minutes)	Waiting Time (Minutes)	Appointment Delay Time (Days)
All Ages			
Under $5,000	25.0	77.9	2.85
$5,000-$9,999	20.7	58.7	3.09
$10,000-$14,999	17.5	45.8	3.73
$15,000 and over	17.1	36.5	3.67
Ratio, highest income to lowest income category	0.68	0.47	1.29
Under 17 Years of Age			
Under $5,000	24.7	94.0	2.12
$5,000-$9,999	20.2	63.2	3.24
$10,000-$14,999	16.9	46.6	3.73
$15,000 and over	17.5	33.4	3.89
Ratio, highest income to lowest income category	0.71	0.36	1.83
Ages 17-44			
Under $5,000	27.0	79.7	3.02
$5,000-$9,999	20.9	60.1	2.89
$10,000-$14,999	16.9	44.9	3.70
$15,000 and over	16.4	37.9	2.93
Ratio, highest income to lowest income category	0.61	0.48	0.97
Ages 45-64			
Under $5,000	25.6	71.8	3.08
$5,000-$9,999	21.8	55.6	2.82
$10,000-$14,999	18.7	45.7	3.39
$15,000 and over	17.8	38.7	4.78
Ratio, highest income to lowest income category	0.70	0.54	1.55
Ages 65 and over			
Under $5,000	23.3	59.9	3.46
$5,000-$9,999	20.0	41.3	3.73
$10,000-$14,999	21.1	45.7	5.67
$15,000 and over	17.3	36.5	2.89
Ratio, highest income to lowest income category	0.74	0.61	0.83

Source: CHAS survey data presented in Frank A. Sloan, "Toward Measures of Equity in the Delivery of Health Care Services," in William R. Rogers (ed.), *Nourishing the Humanistic in Medicine: A Dialogue with the Social Sciences,* Pittsburgh, Pennsylvania: University of Pittsburgh Press (forthcoming), 1979.

Note: Table includes all persons in sample.

"flu," whereas, for a physical examination, the value to the patient of having an examination two weeks from the date an appointment is made may be much the same as an examination occurring four or five weeks from that date.

Data from the Health Interview Surveys conducted by the U.S. National Center for Health Statistics show that the proportion of visits involving diagnosis and treatment as opposed to care of a preventive nature—pre- or postnatal visits, general checkups, eye examinations, and immunizations—declines with increases in patient income.[30] On the whole, it is reasonable to suppose that the benefit from obtaining an early appointment is higher for the former than for the latter kind of care. To the extent that the reason for visit varies systematically with patient income, comparisons of appointment delays must be made with some care. Thus, for example, appointment delays may have fallen because visits for preventive care fell, and yet one could mistakenly conclude that access had improved, at least in the appointment delay dimension.

A Micro Study of Patients

Sloan and Steinwald's data came from a survey of Washington, D.C., families conducted by the Institute of Medicine, National Academy of Sciences. Although the sample is not representative of the United States as a whole, it was superior to national data bases existing at the time because appointment data were available for specific visits. The CHAS data identify the "usual" delay; but if Sloan and Steinwald are correct, the concept of a usual delay has little meaning, unless the patient consistently visits the same physician for the same reason.

The authors found that appointment delays are systematically related to diagnosis or reason for visit and that low-income patients visit physicians for more acute illnesses for which delays are shorter. They then investigated the three-way relationship among patient income, choice of site of care—private offices versus clinics (emergency room visits were excluded)—and diagnosis. Appointment delays were found to be longer for persons visiting clinics, and the negative relationship between illness acuteness and appointment delays held for both private office and clinic samples. Within each sample, the effect of patient income on appointment delays tended to be negative; furthermore, incomes of clinic patients were reported to be far below those of patients of private practitioners.

Patient Satisfaction

To our knowledge, all work on the satisfaction dimension of access has been descriptive rather than based on specific analytical models. Yet, such measures have been used in the past, and we report new evidence on satisfaction in chapter 4. Therefore, a few remarks are in order here.

Considering the satisfaction data from Quebec reported in the Canadian studies, table 2-2's comparable data from the 1971 CHAS survey of the United States,[31] and data from the 1976 Medical Access Study reported in a recent Robert Wood Johnson Foundation publication,[32] it is apparent that (1) the vast majority of respondents tend to be satisfied with the care they *personally* receive and (2) on the whole, satisfaction is not systematically related to family income.

Cross-tabulations between process and satisfaction measures have revealed a definite correspondence between the two types of access measures.[33] For example, persons who actually spend less time with a doctor on a per-visit basis tend to be less satisfied with this dimension of care. Even in view of table 2-2 and other evidence, we do not wish to imply that "pockets" of dissatisfaction could not be discovered if one disaggregated the categories included in the tables into finer subgroups. Also, one should not infer from the evidence that the citizenry is satisfied with the health system as it now stands. When asked general questions about satisfaction with the health care system as opposed to satisfaction with care personally received, a desire for change is apparent, and there are systematic patterns by income class.[34]

Implications

This literature review offers several general implications for the present study.

First, access is multidimensional. Each dimension captures a particular aspect or aspects of the delivery of health care services, but may be deficient in others. It is by no means clear that one should develop a single access measure; nor would it be likely that any single index would ever gain sufficient acceptance by policy makers and experts in the field.

Second, commonly accepted access measures do not always point in the same direction. Some access measures rise and others fall in response to a common exogenous stimulus. To gauge whether access has improved or deteriorated, one must look at a whole range of access measures and make specific value judgments as to their relative importance. Then, perhaps, one can make an overall assessment.

Third, the behavior of many, if not most, of the access measures are amenable to formal modeling. Although progress has been made on the underlying theory, empirical research on these issues is still in its infancy. If additional testing reveals that existing theories do not adequately explain behavior, it will be necessary to develop new ones. In this chapter, we have briefly reviewed theoretical and empirical research conducted to date.

Table 2-2
Dissatisfaction with Aspects of Own Medical Care Received, by Family Income
(Percentage)

	Family Income			
Aspect	*Under $5,000*	*$5,000– $9,999*	*$10,000– $14,999*	*$15,000 and Over*
A. Overall quality of the medical care received	8.8	9.2	10.8	6.7
B. Information given to you about what was wrong with you	16.1	17.2	16.8	11.9
C. Information given to you about what you should do at home to treat illness	10.8	10.6	9.8	8.5
D. Concern of doctors for your overall health rather than just for an isolated symptom or disease	12.6	18.5	17.0	13.5
E. Courtesy and consideration shown you by: doctors	7.1	7.7	7.4	5.9
nurses	9.9	11.2	8.2	8.3
F. Follow-up care received after an initial treatment or operation	6.8	8.3	8.7	4.1
G. Waiting time in doctor's offices or clinics	40.9	40.1	37.3	34.6
H. Availability of medical care at night or weekends	40.1	44.8	45.2	42.0
I. Ease and convenience of getting to a doctor from where you live	19.7	14.7	11.2	7.9
J. Out-of-pocket costs of medical care received	37.6	43.6	41.2	30.8

Source: CHAS survey data presented in Frank A. Sloan, "Toward Measures of Equity in the Delivery of Health Care Services," in William R. Rogers (ed.), *Nourishing the Humanistic in Medicine: A Dialogue with the Social Sciences,* Pittsburgh, Pennsylvania: University of Pittsburgh Press (forthcoming), 1979.

Fourth, we have distinguished between macro and micro studies, and short- versus long-run analyses. It is essential to make these distinctions since the nature of the model and the findings themselves often depend on them. For example, in the short run, comparatively few patients may change providers and few providers may vary practice inputs to any meaningful extent.

Fifth, as seen in chapter 1, inflation and recession have a number of subtle impacts, and many of these are just being studied for the first time. Inflationary and recessionary forces potentially affect both demand and supply sides of the physicians' services market and, perhaps more important, expectations play a role. With both schedules shifting and with complex expectational effects, it is literally impossible to deduce the effects of inflation-recession on conceptual grounds alone. The impacts of adverse economic conditions must be determined empirically. Since some of the effects are potentially subtle, it is necessary to use several techniques and data bases, each with its own positive and negative attributes in order to gain an overall balanced impression of the effects of inflation-recession and other exogenous factors on patient access to physicians' services.

Notes

1. See, for example, Frank Sloan and John Lorant, "The Role of Waiting Time: Evidence from Physicians' Practices," *Journal of Business* 50 (October): 486-507, 1977; Frank Sloan and Roger Feldman, "Competition Among Physicians," in Warren Greenberg (ed.), *Competition in the Health Care Sector: Past, Present, and Future,* Proceedings of a Conference Sponsored by the Federal Trade Commission, March 1978, pp. 57-131.

2. Frank Sloan, Jerry Cromwell, and Janet Mitchell, *Private Physicians and Public Programs,* Lexington, Massachusetts: DC Heath-Lexington, 1978.

3. Supply-side studies include the following operations research-oriented papers: Robert B. Fetter and John D. Thompson, "Patients' Waiting Time and Doctors' Idle Time in the Outpatient Setting," *Health Services Research* 1 (Summer):142-153, 1966; *Lancet,* September 11, 1965, pp. 532-533; M.J.B. White and M.C. Pike, "Appointment System in Outpatient Clinics," *Medical Care* 2 (1964):133-144.

4. Ronald Andersen, *A Behavioral Model of Families' Use of Health Services,* Chicago: Center for Health Administration Studies, University of Chicago (Research Series No. 25) 1968; Ronald Andersen, Joanna Kravits, and Odin Anderson, *Two Decades of Health Services: Social Survey Trends in Use and Expenditure,* Cambridge, Massachusetts: Ballinger Publishing Company, 1975.

5. The same problem emerges when micro demand studies are used to project utilization under universal health insurance. Certainly, estimates at the demand response to a reduced out-of-pocket price overstates the actual utilization response, especially in the short run.

6. David E. Rogers and Robert J. Blendon, "The Changing American Health Scene: Sometimes Things Get Better," *Journal of the American Medical Association* 237 (April 18):1710-1714, 1977.

7. Ronald Andersen, Joanna Lion, and Odin Anderson, *Two Decades of Health Services: Social Survey Trends in Use and Expenditure,* Cambridge, Massachusetts: Ballinger Publishing Company, 1976; Karen Davis, "The Impact of Inflation and Unemployment on Health Care of Low-Income Families," in

Michael Zubkoff (ed.), *Health: A Victim or Cause of Inflation?*, New York: Prodist, 1976, pp. 101-111.

8. For comparisons between 1963 and 1970, see Andersen, Lion, and Anderson, *Two Decades of Health Services*; for 1970 comparison, see Lu Ann Aday, "Economic and Noneconomic Barriers to the Use of Needed Medical Services," *Medical Care* 13 (June):447-56, 1975.

9. Lee Benham and Alexandra Benham, "Utilization of Physician Services Across Income Groups, 1963-1970," in Ronald Andersen, et al. (eds.), *Equity in Health Services,* Cambridge, Massachusetts: Ballinger Publishing Company, 1975, pp. 97-194.

10. For this reason, we have not reviewed the simultaneous equation study of the physician services market provided in Victor Fuchs and Maria Kramer, *Determinants of Expenditures for Physicians' Services in the United States, 1948-1968,* Washington: National Center for Health Services Research and Development, 1972. The Fuchs-Kramer results are useful for other purposes, but not for what they imply about the *current* effect of income and insurance on the demand for physicians' services.

11. David Salkever, "Economic Class and Differential Access to Care: Comparisons Among Health Care Systems," *International Journal of Health Services* 5 (summer): 373-395, 1975.

12. See for example Gary S. Becker, "A Theory of the Allocation of Time," *The Economic Journal* 75 (September):493-517, 1965; and Allan C. DeSerpa, "On the Comparative Statics of Time Allocation Theory," *Canadian Journal of Economics* 8 (February):101-111, 1975.

13. Joseph P. Newhouse and Charles E. Phelps, "New Estimates of Price and Elasticities of Medical Care Services," in Richard Rosett (ed.), *The Role of Health Insurance in the Health Services Sector,* New York: National Bureau of Economic Research, 1976, pp. 261-312.

14. Jan Paul Acton, "Demand for Health Care Among the Urban Poor, With Special Emphasis on the Role of Time," in Richard Rosett (ed.), *The Role of Health Insurance in the Health Services Sector,* New York: National Bureau of Economic Research, 1976, pp. 165-207; Acton, "Nonmonetary Factors in the Demand for Medical Services: Some Empirical Evidence," *Journal of Political Economy* 83 (June):595-615, 1975.

15. These results were obtained previously by Becker and Lancaster using somewhat different models. Becker, "A Theory of the Allocation of Time," and Kelvin Lancaster, "A New Approach to Customer Theory," *Journal of Political Economy* 74 (April):132-57, 1966. The Acton studies provide a clearer theoretical statement to the reader who is not very familiar with economic theory. See also Charles E. Phelps and Joseph P. Newhouse, "Coinsurance, the Price of Time, and Demand for Medical Services," *Review of Economics and Statistics* 56 (August):334-42, 1974, for a discussion of the relationship between the price of time and the utilization of health care services.

16. Jan Paul Acton, "Nonmonetary Factors in the Demand for Medical Services: Some Empirical Evidence," 1975, supra, note 14.

17. Jan Paul Acton, "Demand for Health Care Among the Urban Poor, with Special Emphasis on the Role of Time," 1976, supra, note 14.

18. A study by Inman contains estimates of the time cost effect on demand for health services for children. His results suggest that time costs matter. Robert P. Inman, "The Family Provision of Children's Health: An Economic Analysis," in R. Rosett (ed.), *The Role of Health Insurance in the Health Services Sector,* New York: National Bureau of Economic Research, 1976, pp. 215-259. Other studies of the travel time-utilization relationship include Curtis J. Henke, Edward H. Yelin, Mary Lee Ingbar, and Wallace V. Epstein, "The University Rheumatic Disease Clinic: Provider and Patient Perceptions of Cost," *Arthritis and Rheumatism* 20 (2):751-58, March 1977; James Studenski, "The Minimization of Travel Effort as a Delineating Influence for Urban Hospital Service Areas," *International Journal of Health Services* 5 (4):79-93, 1975; G.W. Shannon, K.L. Bashur, and C.A. Metzner, "The Concept of Distance as a Factor in Accessibility and Utilization of Health Care," *Medical Care Review* 26 (2): 143-161, 1979; J.E. Weiss, M.R. Greenlick, "Determinants of Medical Care Utilization: The Effect of Social Class and Distance on Contacts Within the Medical System," *Medical Care* 8 (6):455-463, 1970.

19. Frank Sloan, "The Demand for Physicians' Services in Alternative Practice Settings: A Multiple Logit Analysis," *Quarterly Review of Economics and Business* 18 (Spring):41-61, 1978.

20. U.S. Department of Health, Education, and Welfare, National Center for Health Statistics, *Physician Visits and Interval Since the Last Visit,* (Vital and Health Statistics), data from the *National Health Survey* 10 (75), Washington: U.S. Government Printing Office, 1972.

21. Spyros, Andreopoulos, (ed.) *Primary Care: Where Medicine Fails,* New York: John Wiley, 1974.

22. Philip E. Enterline, et al., "The Distribution of Medical Services Before and After 'Free' Medical Care—The Quebec Experience," *New England Journal of Medicine* 289 (November 29):1174-8, 1973; Philip E. Enterline, et al., "Effects of 'Free' Medical Care on Medical Practice—The Quebec Experience," *New England Journal of Medicine* 288 (May 31):1152-55, 1973; Alison J. McDonald et al., "Physician Service in Montreal Before Universal Health Insurance," *Medical Care* 11 (July-August):269-286, 1973.

23. See Frank Sloan and John Lorant, "The Role of Waiting Time: Evidence from Physicians' Practices," *Journal of Business* 50 (October):486-507, 1977; and Frank Sloan and Bruce Steinwald, "Variations in Appointment Delays for Physician Services: Theory and Empirical Evidence," *Policy Sciences* (forthcoming).

24. More recent information on the Quebec experience under Medicare may be found in Philip Held et al., *A Study of the Responses of Canadian*

Physicians to the Introduction of Universal Medical Care Insurance: The First Five Years in Quebec, Final Report on Contract No. HRA 230-75-0167 between U.S. Department of Health, Education, and Welfare and Mathematica Policy Research, Inc.

25. See Sloan and Lorant, "The Role of Waiting Time" and Sloan and Steinwald, "Variations in Appointment Delays."

26. Sloan and Lorant, "The Role of Waiting Time."

27. Frank Sloan and John Lorant, "The Allocation of Physicians' Services: Evidence on Length-of-Visit," *Quarterly Review of Economics and Business* 16 (Autumn):85–103, 1976.

28. See, for example, studies by Reinhardt: Uwe E. Reinhardt, "A Product Function for Physician Services," *Review of Economics and Statistics* 54 (February):55–66, 1972; Uwe E. Reinhardt, *Physician Productivity and the Demand for Health Manpower,* Cambridge, Massachusetts: Ballinger Publishing Company, 1975.

29. Sloan and Steinwald, "Variations in Appointment Delays."

30. U.S. Department of Health, Education, and Welfare, National Center for Health Statistics, *Physician Visits and Interval Since the Last Visit, United States, 1969,* (Vital and Health Statistics), data from the *National Health Survey* 10 (75), Washington: U.S. Government Printing Office, 1972.

31. The CHAS survey data are presented in: Frank A. Sloan, "Toward Measures of Equity in the Delivery of Health Care Services," in William R. Rogers (ed.), *Nourishing the Humanistic in Medicine: A Dialogue with the Social Sciences,* Pittsburgh, Pennsylvania: University of Pittsburgh Press (forthcoming) 1979.

32. The Robert Wood Johnson Foundation, *Special Report on Access—America's Health Care System: A Comprehensive Portrait,* Princeton, New Jersey, 1978.

33. The CHAS survey evidence is presented in Sloan, "Toward Measures of Equity."

34. Sloan, "Toward Measures of Equity"; The Robert Wood Johnson Foundation, "Special Report on Access."

3

Utilization of Physicians' Services: A Time-Series Analysis

Utilization of physicians' services is one dimension of access to ambulatory care among three to be assessed in this study. In this chapter, we use cross-tabular as well as multivariate procedures to investigate the impact of adverse economic conditions on utilization of physicians' services, both in the aggregate and by site of care. Whereas the cross-tabulations offer the opportunity to obtain a quick, broad appraisal of the impact of rising inflation and rising unemployment on utilization, the multivariate analysis provides a more detailed perspective of underlying behavioral relationships. Multivariate analysis allows us to better isolate the impacts of particular factors on our access measures.

The primary data source for the analysis outlined in this chapter is a set of unpublished tabulations based on Health Interview Surveys (HIS) conducted annually by the National Center for Health Statistics (NCHS). The NCHS has provided us with tabulations for the years 1969 through 1975. Analysis of the years 1969–1975 permits an assessment of utilization patterns both before and during the worst inflation-recession period in recent history. The Health Interview Survey is part of the National Health Survey that has been conducted regularly since 1957. From this survey, we were able to obtain detailed information on number and site of physician visits as well as the occurrence and severity of illness and disability.

At the onset of our discussion, we review these data and attempt to draw inferences regarding the impact of adverse economic conditions on access to ambulatory care. Although we are able to identify several secular trends, no cyclical trends are immediately obvious. The secular improvement in access is consistent with findings of other studies noted in chapter 2. In addition, we consider the utilization dimensions of the access to care by employment status. Again we are unable to identify any cyclical fluctuations, but we are able to postulate interesting hypotheses concerning the effect of employment status on health.

In order to further investigate implications suggested by these data, we specify a dynamic model of physicians' services utilization that we estimate using multiple regression analysis. In this analysis, we merge HIS data with additional socioeconomic data representing access determinants. The results of this analysis provide insights into the relative importance of each of these determinants; furthermore, we find a link between inflation-recession and physicians' services utilization.

We conclude chapter 3 with a discussion of our findings in relationship to previous research. Throughout this discussion, we attempt to focus on the relevant policy implications of our findings.

Descriptive Analysis

The Mean Number of Physician Visits

The number of physician visits incorporates both the number of initial contacts and return visits to a physician. Visits at all sites are included. As seen in table 3-1, in 1975 there were, on the average, slightly over five visits to a physician per person overall nationally (including those who did not see a physician at all). Of all age groups, children (under age 17) had the fewest visits to the physician on the average; older adults (age 65-74) and the elderly (age 75+) had the most visits overall.

On a nationwide basis, the number of physician visits increased by 21.4 percent during the period 1969 through 1975. The youngest (under age 17) group made striking gains in utilization compared to the older groups. According to the means shown in table 3-1, visits for those under age 17 increased 16.6 percent; comparable rates of increase for those aged 65-74 and those over age 75 were 8.1 percent and 6.4 percent. From table 3-1, one may infer that visits per person per year for all ages were generally increasing during the early and mid-1970s and seem to be relatively insensitive to worsening conditions in the economy.

A consideration of health status-adjusted utilization patterns leads to a substantially different utilization pattern from that implied above. Measures of health status in this chapter are restricted-activity days and bed-disability days.[1] Comparing all age categories, children, not surprisingly, have the highest number of visits per restricted-activity day and per bed-disability day; persons age 75 and older have the lowest health-adjusted utilization rate.[2]

In contrast to the visit series, neither a secular trend nor a cyclical pattern is evident from the health status-adjusted visit data. Over the entire period, 1969 through 1975, health-adjusted physician utilization remained fairly constant. There is no clear relationship exhibited between visits per restricted-activity day or visits per bed-disability day and adverse economic conditions.

If we consider the trends in the utilization of physicians' services from a more disaggregated perspective, as table 3-2 allows one to do, it is apparent that, since the late 1960s, the poor have made substantial gains relative to the middle and upper income groups. Overall the number of mean physician visits increased

Table 3-1
Trends in Physician Visits

Year	All Ages	<17	17–24	25–44	45–64	65–74	75+
Physician Visits Per Person and Year							
1969	4.2	3.6	4.0	4.3	4.7	6.1	6.2
1970	4.6	3.9	4.6	4.6	5.2	6.0	6.7
1971	4.9	4.2	4.9	4.8	5.4	6.4	7.2
1972	5.0	4.1	4.9	5.0	5.5	6.6	7.4
1973	5.0	4.2	4.9	5.1	5.5	6.5	6.6
1974	4.9	4.1	4.5	5.0	5.5	6.9	6.5
1975	5.1	4.2	4.8	5.1	5.6	6.6	6.6
Visits Per Restricted-Activity Day							
1969	0.29	0.36	0.44	0.33	0.23	0.20	0.16
1970	0.32	0.41	0.47	0.34	0.26	0.21	0.19
1971	0.31	0.39	0.47	0.36	0.26	0.22	0.17
1972	0.30	0.38	0.44	0.34	0.24	0.21	0.17
1973	0.30	0.39	0.42	0.35	0.24	0.21	0.17
1974	0.29	0.39	0.40	0.34	0.23	0.19	0.16
1975	0.28	0.39	0.39	0.32	0.23	0.19	0.14
Visits Per Bed-Disability Day							
1969	0.70	0.76	1.0	0.84	0.62	0.55	0.38
1970	0.76	0.89	1.0	0.89	0.69	0.48	0.41
1971	0.81	0.88	1.1	0.89	0.73	0.64	0.39
1972	0.77	0.89	1.0	0.89	0.70	0.58	0.39
1973	0.79	0.93	0.94	0.93	0.70	0.60	0.39
1974	0.74	0.86	0.99	0.86	0.65	0.54	0.38
1975	0.77	0.96	0.94	0.87	0.69	0.64	0.38

Source: U.S. Department of Health, Education, and Welfare, National Center for Health Statistics, "Health Interview Surveys" (unpublished data), 1975.

21.4 percent; in the lowest income group visits increased 30.4 percent; and in the highest income group visits increased by 13.9 percent.

Although the data in table 3-2 give solid support to the contention that the poor's access to physician visits improved over the time period 1969 through 1975, the improvements were not shared equally by all persons. Children under age 17 and persons over age 65 experienced the largest and smallest gains, respectively.

Considering the relationship of family size and physician use, the data suggest that persons in large families tended to have lower levels of use than persons in small families. As seen in table 3-2, the number of physician visits per child per year in one- to two-person families was, on the average, 6.5 in 1975. By contrast, for families of seven or more persons, the mean was 2.7 visits per child. Controlling for age, a clear inverse relationship between family size and the physician utilization of child family members is apparent; the same influence

Table 3-2
Physician Visits by Age, Family Size, and Income

Year	All Sizes All Income	All Sizes <$5,000	All Sizes $5,000-$9,999	All Sizes >$10,000	1-2 Persons All Income	1-2 Persons <$5,000	1-2 Persons $5,000-$9,999	1-2 Persons >$10,000	3-4 Persons All Income	3-4 Persons <$5,000	3-4 Persons $5,000-$9,999	3-4 Persons >$10,000	5-6 Persons All Income	5-6 Persons <$5,000	5-6 Persons $5,000-$9,999	5-6 Persons >$10,000	7+ Persons All Income	7+ Persons <$5,000	7+ Persons $5,000-$9,999	7+ Persons >$10,000
All Ages																				
1969	4.2	4.6	4.0	4.3	5.3	6.0	5.2	5.2	4.5	4.4	4.4	4.7	3.7	3.4	3.5	4.1	2.4	2.3	2.4	2.6
1970	4.6	5.0	4.4	4.7	5.8	5.9	6.0	5.7	4.8	4.8	4.5	5.0	4.0	3.8	3.7	4.3	3.0	3.0	2.6	3.5
1971	4.9	5.6	4.7	4.9	6.1	6.7	5.8	6.1	5.2	5.5	5.1	5.3	4.1	3.9	3.9	4.3	3.2	3.5	2.7	3.4
1972	5.0	5.6	4.8	4.9	6.1	6.7	5.5	6.0	5.1	5.2	5.2	5.2	4.2	4.0	3.9	4.5	3.1	2.8	3.2	3.1
1973	5.0	5.7	4.8	5.0	6.0	6.8	6.1	5.7	5.3	5.5	4.9	5.5	4.2	4.2	3.8	4.4	3.1	3.2	3.5	3.0
1974	5.0	5.6	5.0	4.8	6.1	6.1	6.4	5.8	5.0	5.1	4.9	5.5	4.2	3.8	3.7	4.4	3.2	3.4	2.7	3.0
1975	5.1	6.0	5.2	4.9	6.1	6.9	6.3	5.8	5.2	5.6	5.3	5.2	4.0	n.a.	n.a.	n.a.	n.a.	n.a.	n.a.	n.a.
Children Under 17																				
1969	3.6	2.8	3.4	4.2	5.2	5.7	5.0	4.5	4.8	4.1	4.7	5.3	3.4	2.4	3.1	4.1	2.0	1.3	2.0	2.4
1970	3.9	3.4	3.6	4.3	6.1	6.5	5.6	6.9	5.0	4.0	4.9	5.3	3.6	2.9	3.1	4.2	2.5	2.3	2.3	2.9
1971	4.2	3.8	3.9	4.6	6.7	7.6	6.4	4.3	5.5	4.6	5.4	6.0	3.7	2.8	3.5	4.2	2.6	2.6	2.2	3.0
1972	4.1	3.6	3.9	4.4	6.1	6.1	4.8	6.7	5.3	4.6	5.3	5.7	3.7	3.2	3.2	4.1	2.4	2.1	2.5	2.4
1973	4.2	3.9	3.8	4.5	6.2	7.3	4.9	3.6	5.3	4.2	4.8	5.8	3.7	3.1	3.1	4.0	2.6	2.3	2.9	2.5
1974	4.1	3.7	3.7	4.5	5.4	5.4	6.2	4.7	5.2	4.0	4.8	5.6	3.6	2.8	3.2	3.9	2.7	2.8	2.0	3.0
1975	4.3	4.6	3.9	4.4	6.5	7.6	6.2	5.9	5.3	5.0	5.3	5.4	3.7	n.a.	n.a.	n.a.	n.a.	n.a.	n.a.	n.a.
Adults 25-64																				
1969	4.5	5.3	4.2	4.4	4.9	5.4	7.0	4.7	4.3	4.8	4.1	4.5	4.2	5.0	4.0	4.1	3.5	4.7	3.5	3.1
1970	5.2	5.1	4.6	4.9	5.4	5.3	5.6	5.4	4.6	5.9	4.2	4.7	4.6	5.4	4.4	4.5	4.4	5.3	3.4	5.1
1971	5.1	6.1	5.0	5.0	5.7	6.6	5.4	5.8	5.0	5.9	4.9	5.0	4.5	5.0	4.5	4.5	4.4	6.6	3.7	4.1
1972	5.2	6.1	5.0	5.2	5.6	6.0	5.2	5.8	5.0	6.2	5.0	4.9	5.1	6.0	4.8	5.2	4.6	4.8	4.6	4.4
1973	5.3	6.6	5.0	5.3	5.6	7.1	5.6	5.5	5.3	6.6	4.9	5.3	4.9	6.4	4.8	5.0	4.3	6.1	4.7	4.0
1974	5.2	6.6	5.5	5.0	5.8	6.7	5.9	5.6	5.1	6.6	5.5	4.9	4.5	5.8	4.3	4.5	4.3	4.7	4.5	3.9
1975	5.3	7.1	5.4	5.1	5.7	7.0	5.7	5.6	5.3	7.0	5.2	5.2	n.a.	n.a.	n.a.	n.a.	n.a.	n.a.	n.a.	n.a.
Adults 65 and Over																				
1967	6.1	6.1	5.8	7.5	6.2	6.3	5.8	8.0	6.0	5.9	6.2	6.7	5.5	4.0	4.4	7.3	4.7	6.9	3.5	4.0
1970	6.3	6.1	6.3	7.4	6.4	6.4	6.9	6.7	6.3	5.7	5.3	8.2	7.0	7.1	6.0	8.0	4.0	4.0	2.3	5.5
1971	6.7	6.7	6.3	7.5	6.6	6.5	6.2	8.3	6.1	6.3	5.9	6.4	7.0	10.2	7.0	7.0	7.6	4.2	14.5	5.8
1972	6.9	7.1	6.7	6.7	6.8	7.1	6.2	6.5	6.6	5.9	7.6	7.1	6.7	6.1	9.2	5.5	5.5	5.7	6.4	5.7
1973	6.5	6.6	6.5	7.1	6.7	6.8	6.2	7.1	6.7	5.9	5.3	7.6	5.8	7.1	6.0	6.1	5.9	7.0	8.3	5.7
1974	6.7	6.3	6.8	7.7	6.7	6.0	6.8	7.9	6.4	5.0	6.9	6.9	10.2	8.3	13.9	9.6	8.6	10.7	6.9	8.8
1975	6.6	6.5	6.1	6.6	6.8	7.0	7.2	6.6	6.2	4.5	7.9	6.6	n.a.	n.a.	n.a.	n.a.	n.a.	n.a.	n.a.	n.a.

Source: U.S. Department of Health, Education, and Welfare, National Center for Health Statistics, Health Interview Surveys (unpublished data), 1975.
n.a. = data not available

of family size on the utilization of adult family members is evident, but this latter pattern is less clear.

Combining income with family size, the largest discrepancies in children's physician contact by family size by 1975 was within middle-income families. A 67 percent difference separated large and small families in the middle-income group. But for low-income families the gap was 48 percent, and for high-income families the difference is only 36 percent. These numbers imply that the marginal effect of another family member (and a corresponding decrease in per capita income) was greatest for members of the middle class.

Moreover, in the late 1960s, the largest discrepancies in children's physician contact by family size were within the low-income group. During the period 1969-1975, however, this discrepancy narrowed. In fact, during these years, large families increased their utilization of physician services at a greater rate than small families and, as mentioned earlier, the low-income group increased their utilization more than the middle- and high-income groups. In contrast to the above, cyclical trends pertaining to physician utilization by family size and income are not as easily identified.

The tabulations in table 3-2 imply that the association between family size and adults' use of physicians' services is low. The incidence of disease varies systematically by income class. A study by Bentkover and Sanders reported an inverse relationship between income level and reported activity limitation;[3] the average number of days of activity limitation per capita was seen to be higher for low-income individuals in every year from 1969 through 1975.

We have prepared tables in a format similar to table 3-2, but replacing visits by visits per restricted-activity day and per bed-disability day.[4] From these tables, it is apparent that the difference in health-adjusted physician utilization associated with family size is much smaller than the corresponding difference in the unadjusted utilization rates. As discussed previously, there was a 140 percent difference in children's utilization rates between very small and very large families. This difference is reduced to approximately 35 percent when health status is held constant.

When age is held constant, the most significant inverse relationship between family size and utilization is obtained for children. Contrary to our previous finding, when adjusted rates of physician utilization are considered, the largest disparity in children's utilization by family size is within high-income families, although the differences between disparities within the high-income group and the middle-income group is much smaller than noted earlier.

Consistent with our foregoing conclusions, the tabulations suggest that health-adjusted physician utilization rates increased more for large families than for small families during the seven-year period. Furthermore, when one compares rates of increased utilization by income group, it is evident that the high-income group experienced the smallest percentage increase. Contrary to patterns in the unadjusted utilization tabulations, the health-adjusted utilization information indicates that the middle income group experienced the largest increase.

Physician Visits by Site of Care

Table 3-3 reveals that nearly 13 percent of all physician visits occurred in an outpatient clinic or emergency room, 12.5 percent of all visits were "telephone visits," and slightly less than one percent of total visits were home visits. Whereas all persons except the very old were apt to use the outpatient clinic and emergency room, the aged were more than six times as likely to receive home care than was the population at large. Individuals between the ages of 25 and 44 were least likely to receive care at home. Telephone visits are most commonly associated with children's health problems and least commonly associated with older persons' ailments.

Table 3-3
Site of Care by Age and Year as a Percentage of Total Visits

Year	All Ages	<17	17-24	25-44	45-64	65-74	75+
Outpatient clinic and emergency room							
1969	10.3	11.9	11.2	11.9	8.8	5.9	6.3
1970	10.6	12.2	11.2	9.9	10.7	8.5	6.3
1971	10.2	11.4	12.7	9.4	10.1	7.9	4.5
1972	10.9	11.7	12.7	10.6	11.1	8.5	6.4
1973	10.7	11.8	12.8	10.0	10.1	8.5	8.2
1974	11.9	12.3	15.9	12.2	10.7	7.8	8.3
1975	12.9	14.6	14.6	13.3	12.1	10.6	6.3
Home visits							
1969	2.3	1.6	0.9	1.1	1.9	4.7	13.6
1970	2.0	0.7	0.6	1.1	2.0	5.4	11.5
1971	1.7	0.7	0.4	0.7	1.8	3.9	11.3
1972	1.4	0.9	0.8	0.7	0.6	3.2	9.2
1973	1.4	1.6	0.7	0.5	0.8	2.4	7.8
1974	1.1	0.7	0.3	0.6	0.9	2.2	7.8
1975	0.8	0.5	0.3	0.2	0.7	1.0	6.2
Telephone visits							
1969	12.0	19.3	8.7	10.5	7.8	9.0	8.5
1970	12.2	17.8	9.2	11.2	9.3	9.4	10.1
1971	13.3	20.3	10.2	11.7	10.1	9.2	10.7
1972	12.6	19.7	10.7	11.5	8.8	10.1	9.2
1973	12.7	18.6	10.1	12.3	9.9	9.5	9.3
1974	12.3	18.5	9.3	12.0	9.2	8.6	10.3
1975	12.5	17.7	12.2	12.2	9.7	8.3	8.8

Source: Department of Health, Education, and Welfare, National Center for Health Statistics, Health Interview Surveys (unpublished data), 1975.

Regarding the site of care, several secular trends are apparent. Most noteworthy are the tendencies for outpatient clinic and emergency room visits as a percentage of total visits to increase and home visits to decrease. Several factors may account for the trend. First, it is frequently asserted by physicians that the secular decline in home visits reflects the increased technical sophistication of medicine. Adequate medical care can no longer be delivered in the home. An alternative explanation considers home visits as an amenity. During adverse times, such as during the Great Depression of the 1930s, physicians made house calls as a means of generating business; home visits were a "loss leader" of sorts. Given the prosperity of the post-World War II years and more widespread insurance coverage for physicians' services, physicians no longer found it as necessary to provide this amenity. These two explanations, of course, are not mutually exclusive. But it should be noted that the recession of 1974–1975 did not reverse the downward trend in home visits. Finally, the increase in the use of the hospital on an outpatient basis may be attributed in part to the substantial increase in the past decade in the number of hospital-based physicians, many of whom are graduates of foreign medical schools.

In contrast to home and telephone visits, the share of total visits taking place in hospital outpatient clinics and emergency rooms rose substantially in 1975. The possibility that the increase is largely attributable to the recession certainly cannot be ruled out. However, as seen in table 3–4, the outpatient department-emergency room percentages increased about as often in the $10,000 and over income class as in the $5,000 and under class. If the recession caused individuals to depend more on the hospital as a source of ambulatory care, the effect is not more apparent for the poor than for the nonpoor.

Utilization and Employment Status

A tentative estimate of the differences in the access to care can be obtained from comparisons between utilization and employment status. Although this method is straightforward, it is likely to yield biased estimates of the differences to the extent that employed persons are systematically different from unemployed persons. Table 3-5 probably overestimates the *impact* of unemployment on these access variables. Nevertheless, as a first approximation, the identification of general, albeit biased, tendencies in the differences may be useful.

The most recent (1975) data indicate that the unemployed have 34 percent more physician visits per person, between 50 and 60 percent fewer health-adjusted physician visits, and are only one percent more likely to have seen a physician within the last twelve months. When site of care is considered, it is apparent that the unemployed have a greater percentage of outpatient clinic, emergency room, and telephone visits than the employed; presumably, the employed are receiving more private, office-based care.

Table 3-4
Outpatient, Clinic, and Emergency Room Visits as a Percentage of Total Value

	All Sizes				1-2 Persons				3-4 Persons				5-6 Persons				7+ Persons			
Year	All In-come	<$5,000	$5,000-$9,999	>$10,000	All In-come	<$5,000	$5,000-$9,999	>$10,000	All In-come	<$5,000	$5,000-$9,999	>$10,000	All In-come	<$5,000	$5,000-$9,999	>$10,000	All In-come	<$5,000	$5,000-$9,999	>$10,000
Children under 17																				
1969	11.9	23.0	12.2	7.7	26.4	23.9	27.5	35.3	11.7	20.7	13.0	7.0	10.8	25.9	10.8	7.3	13.2	25.2	11.0	10.6
1970	12.2	22.5	13.2	8.2	23.2	25.4	n.a.	n.a.	10.6	19.7	11.4	8.5	11.8	28.4	13.0	7.4	16.3	23.6	17.5	10.2
1971	11.4	21.9	13.3	6.9	21.0	23.3	17.3	20.9	9.8	21.6	9.9	6.0	11.6	25.5	14.6	7.8	14.7	18.0	23.0	6.8
1972	11.7	18.6	13.7	8.9	21.6	27.6	18.7	19.4	9.9	17.2	10.6	7.7	11.4	15.2	15.3	9.2	17.7	23.2	21.6	5.8
1973	11.8	21.2	12.9	8.9	18.8	27.2	9.0	n.a.	10.1	20.2	11.9	7.5	12.0	23.6	12.0	9.9	17.2	26.2	18.3	12.4
1974	12.3	25.3	15.3	9.1	12.1	16.8	6.2	11.2	10.6	24.6	13.2	7.6	12.3	28.2	17.2	9.6	19.8	30.9	24.6	14.6
1975	14.5	23.1	20.7	10.4	20.7	26.0	14.4	n.a.	13.2	21.7	19.2	9.2	14.4	n.a.	n.a.	n.a.	n.a.	n.a.	n.a.	n.a.
Adults 25-64																				
1969	10.4	15.3	9.2	8.9	8.0	10.6	4.5	7.8	9.6	18.8	9.3	7.4	12.7	16.8	9.6	12.7	13.4	6.8	n.a.	n.a.
1970	10.3	17.7	10.9	7.5	9.8	13.2	11.2	7.1	10.4	21.7	10.6	8.2	10.5	16.8	12.5	6.6	11.8	n.a.	12.3	9.3
1971	9.8	16.4	10.2	13.9	8.6	13.1	9.2	6.4	9.4	16.4	10.8	7.1	8.9	15.7	7.0	8.5	11.9	n.a.	14.4	6.4
1972	10.8	17.7	11.5	8.2	10.4	16.7	10.1	8.3	9.7	17.3	11.5	7.5	10.5	16.0	10.6	9.0	12.6	n.a.	17.8	10.3
1973	10.1	16.0	11.0	8.3	9.4	16.6	9.1	7.2	9.3	12.4	11.3	7.8	11.0	21.4	8.8	10.1	14.6	n.a.	n.a.	10.6
1974	11.5	17.5	12.5	9.8	10.6	12.5	12.3	9.5	11.4	23.7	11.3	9.5	12.2	21.8	17.3	10.4	13.6	n.a.	18.1	11.7
1975	12.7	19.7	15.0	10.4	11.4	12.8	11.3	11.2	11.6	20.4	15.9	9.4	n.a.	n.a.	n.a.	n.a.	n.a.	n.a.	n.a.	n.a.
Adults 65 and Over																				
1969	6.0	6.7	4.1	5.9	5.4	5.0	5.4	n.a.	3.5	n.a.	n.a.	6.3	6.2	n.a.	n.a.	9.7	17.7	28.2	n.a.	n.a.
1970	7.7	7.7	5.6	8.5	6.7	7.9	4.5	6.8	10.0	3.0	7.7	15.2	10.2	n.a.	15.8	3.7	n.a.	n.a.	n.a.	n.a.
1971	6.5	7.1	6.5	5.0	7.2	7.0	8.1	7.0	4.6	7.1	n.a.	2.1	6.6	15.8	n.a.	n.a.	8.1	n.a.	n.a.	n.a.
1972	7.7	8.7	7.5	4.5	6.8	8.2	6.0	2.4	4.4	2.9	5.8	n.a.	8.3	n.a.	20.7	n.a.	12.0	n.a.	n.a.	n.a.
1973	8.4	8.3	6.2	12.5	7.4	6.7	6.0	13.1	11.9	14.9	8.4	13.9	12.0	41.0	n.a.	10.0	n.a.	n.a.	n.a.	n.a.
1974	8.7	9.3	10.1	7.0	9.0	10.8	10.8	6.1	7.5	7.2	7.0	5.7	16.0	27.6	n.a.	9.9	12.9	27.9	n.a.	11.8
1975	9.0	8.4	9.4	9.5	9.1	8.1	10.2	10.2	8.4	11.2	7.4	8.4	n.a.	n.a.	n.a.	n.a.	n.a.	n.a.	n.a.	n.a.

Source: Department of Health, Education, and Welfare, National Center for Health Statistics, Health Interview Surveys (unpublished data), 1975.
n.a. = data not available.

Table 3–5
Trends in Physician Visits by Employment Status (Adults 25–64)

Year	Currently Employed	Currently Unemployed
Physician visits per person, per year		
1969	3.8	7.4
1970	4.2	7.4
1971	4.3	7.6
1972	4.4	7.4
1973	4.4	8.9
1974	4.3	8.6
1975	4.4	5.9
Visits per restricted activity day		
1969	.35	.14
1970	.39	.12
1971	.39	.16
1972	.38	.16
1973	.37	.17
1974	.37	.17
1975	.35	.17
Visits per bed disability day		
1969	.96	.33
1970	1.1	.39
1971	1.1	.48
1972	1.1	.44
1973	1.1	.49
1974	1.1	.50
1975	1.1	.47
Percentage of visits to outpatient clinics and emergency rooms		
1969	9.7	12.0
1970	9.5	n.a.
1971	8.0	9.3
1972	10.0	16.3
1973	8.9	8.4
1974	10.9	10.6
1975	10.9	15.2
Percentage of home visits		
1969	1.2	n.a.
1970	1.1	3.9
1971	1.2	1.2
1972	0.7	0.5
1973	0.5	n.a.
1974	0.7	0.8
1975	0.1	0.5
Percentage of telephone visits		
1969	7.9	8.9
1970	9.7	13.5
1971	10.1	11.3
1972	9.3	11.4
1973	10.5	12.9
1974	10.1	11.6
1975	10.8	10.8

Source: Department of Health, Education, and Welfare, National Center for Health Statistics, Health Interview Surveys (unpublished data), 1975.

n.a. = data not available

These trends have remained fairly constant over time. The unemployed typically have had a higher mean number of physician visits per year, a lower mean number of adjusted physician visits per year, and higher utilization rates of outpatient, emergency room, and telephone services.

Multivariate Analysis

The highly aggregated data in the preceding tables do not show sufficient cyclical variation in order to allow us to gain a detailed perspective on the relationship between access to medical care and adverse economic conditions prevailing in 1974-1975. As indicated in chapter 1, economic theory does not offer a prediction about the effects of inflation on consumption. Reasons can be given for positive and negative effects. The net impact of inflation on the utilization of physicians' services must be settled on an empirical basis.

In this section, we present a model to serve as a basis of additional analysis of the utilization dimension of access. The specification is somewhat limited by the fact that the sample consists of only twenty-eight quarterly observations, covering the years 1969-1975. The observational unit for this analysis is the entire United States. Separate regressions are estimated for different age groups; regressions combining all age groups are also presented.

Specification of the Model

We suggest three propositions in order to capture the crucial features of the market for the physician services: (1) the demand for physicians' services is expected to be primarily related to predisposing variables—age and habit persistence, enabling variables—income, level of health insurance coverage, availability of physician services, inflation, and unemployment, and need or health status variables; (2) the supply side can *as a first approximation* be represented by the patient care-physician-population ratio;[5] and (3) health status is a function of age, inflation, unemployment, and seasonal effects.

The above propositions imply the following equations:

$$DVP_{it} = \alpha_0 + \alpha_1 YRP_t + \alpha_2 MDSP_t + \alpha_3 REXP_t + \alpha_4 CPIC_t + \alpha_5 U_t$$
$$+ \alpha_6 HS_t + \alpha_7 DVP_{i,\,t-1} \tag{3.1}$$

$$HS_{it} = \beta_0 + \beta_1 CPIC_t + \beta_2 U_t + \beta_3 Q_2 + \beta_4 Q_3$$
$$+ \beta_5 Q_4 \tag{3.2}$$

where

DVP_{it} = the mean number of physician visits per person in age group i in period t;

YRP_t = real per capita income in period t;

$MDSP_t$ = the nonfederal patient care physician ratio in period t;

$REXP_t$ = the proportion of physician fees paid by third parties in period t;

$CPIC_t$ = the inflation rate in period t;

U_t = the unemployment rate in period t;

HS_{it} = the health status of age group i in period t;

$DVP_{i,\,t-1}$ = the mean number of physician visits per person in age group i in period $t-1$;

Q_2, Q_3, Q_4 = the second, third, and fourth quarters of the year.

There are two relationships, one explaining the utilization of physician services in terms of both demand and supply influences (a reduced form) and the other explaining health status. It is convenient to describe the model by considering first the health status relationship and then the behavioral relationship pertaining to physicians' services utilization.

The variables that are likely to affect health status are age, income, prevailing economic conditions, seasonality, and prior health status. Because the marginal effect (slope) on health status of each variable is likely to vary by age, and since other aspects of the underlying structure are not necessarily identical, we controlled for age by splitting our sample into age subsamples. A priori, for example, we might expect that prevailing economic conditions have a greater effect on the health status of adults than on the health status of children because adults are more likely to experience the emotional and resulting physical repercussions of adverse economic conditions. Thus, our model is specified in accordance with our expectation that the health status relation varies with age.

Furthermore, health status is expected to vary inversely with adverse economic conditions. This hypothesized relationship receives support from previous research by Brenner.[6] We expect that seasonal factors are also likely to influence our measures of health status. Respiratory diseases in particular are more common in winter.

Turning to the utilization of physician services, it is again likely that there are sufficient differences among age groups to estimate separate regressions for each age group. Our utilization equation incorporates both exogenous demand and supply factors. Demand for physicians' services is expected to vary directly with the level of real per capita income, the proportion of expenditures on physicians' services covered by third parties, unemployment and inflation rates, and health status. Health status is represented alternatively as restricted-activity days and bed-disability days.

Supply is represented by the ratio of nonfederal patient-care physicians to population. This is clearly a naive specification of the supply side. Unfortunately, we are limited by the number of supply variables available on a time-series basis as well as the number of explanatory variables that can be included in a regression based on twenty-eight observations. Ideally, we would have wanted to include factor price measures in the equation—prices of nonphysician personnel, and measures of the physician's shadow wage, such as his age, the number of children in his family, and his property income.

Studies of demand for health services often include measures of physician availability; in fact, some authors, such as Fuchs and Kramer,[7] have justified inclusion of these supply variables as demand determinants on grounds that the supply of doctors creates its own demand. Whether or not supply-created demand is important empirically is beyond the scope of our study. Both the traditional economist's model of supply and demand and the supply-created demand model require that a measure of physician availability be included in an utilization equation such as 3.1. According to both views, an increase in the physician-population ratio is predicted to boost utilization.[8]

A lagged dependent variable is included as an explanatory variable to measure short- versus long-term responses to changes in the exogenous variables. Each of the regression parameters of 3.1, α_1 through α_6, depict short-run effects of changes in the explanatory variables. To solve for the long-run responses, we set $DVP_{i,\,t-1}$ equal to DVP_{it}. Then

$$DVP_{it}(1 - \alpha_7) = \alpha_0 + \alpha_1 YRP_t + \alpha_2 MDSP_t + \alpha_3 REXP_t$$
$$+ \alpha_4 CPIC_t + \alpha_5 U_t + \alpha_6 HS_t \qquad (3.3)$$

or

$$DVP_{it} = \frac{\alpha_0}{1 - \alpha_7} + \frac{\alpha_1}{1 - \alpha_7} YRP_t + \frac{\alpha_2}{1 - \alpha_7} MDSP_t + \frac{\alpha_3}{1 - \alpha_7} REXP_t$$
$$+ \frac{\alpha_4}{1 - \alpha_7} CPIC_t + \frac{\alpha_5}{1 - \alpha_7} U_t + \frac{\alpha_6}{1 - \alpha_7} HS_t \qquad (3.4)$$

The coefficients of equation 3.4, $\dfrac{\alpha_i}{1 - \alpha_7}$, $i = 0, 6$, give the long-run responses to changes in the explanatory variables.

Whereas equation 3.1, as specified, contains no current endogenous variables found within the structural form of those two equations, it does contain an endogenous variable from another structural equation, namely, the health status equation. Equation 3.1 gives the *direct effects* of inflation and unemployment on utilization, but inflation and unemployment may also have *indirect* effects on utilization via their influence on health status. To gauge the *total effects* of these explanatory variables on utilization, we substitute equation 3.2 into 3.1, obtaining:

$$
\begin{aligned}
DVP_{it} = {} & \alpha_0 + \alpha_1 YRP_t + \alpha_2 MDSP_t + \alpha_3 REXP_t \\
& + (\alpha_4 + \alpha_6 \beta_1) CPIC_t + (\alpha_5 + \alpha_6 \beta_2) U_t \\
& + \alpha_6 (\beta_0 + \beta_3 Q_2 + \beta_4 Q_3 + \beta_5 Q_4) \\
& + \alpha_7 DVP_{i,\,t-1}
\end{aligned}
\tag{3.5}
$$

From equation 3.5, it is evident that the *total, short-run* impacts of *CPIC* and *U* are $(\alpha_4 + \alpha_6 \beta_1)$ and $(\alpha_5 + \alpha_6 \beta_2)$, respectively. In this context, the short-run impact is the impact occurring in the first quarter. Accordingly, if there is a one percent change in the unemployment rate, doctor visits would change by $(\alpha_5 + \alpha_6 \beta_2)$ in the first quarter. A corresponding change in the inflation rate would change doctor visits by $(\alpha_4 + \alpha_6 \beta_1)$. Estimates of the *total, long-run effects* of inflation and unemployment may be readily derived by substituting equation 3.2 into equation 3.4 and solving. As the model is specified, the full effect would only take place after a very large number (an infinite number) of quarters. The major part of the long-run effect, however, is likely to occur after a few quarters. Given an estimate of the parameter associated with the lagged dependent variable, it is possible to calculate the proportion of the long-run effect that has been realized, quarter by quarter.

An alternative to the above dynamic specification is a static model with the following structure:

$$
\begin{aligned}
DVP_t = {} & \alpha_0 + \alpha_1 YRP_t + \alpha_2 MDSP_t + \alpha_3 REXP_t + \alpha_4 CPIC_t \\
& + \alpha_5 U_t + \alpha_6 HS_t
\end{aligned}
\tag{3.6}
$$

$$
\begin{aligned}
HS_t = {} & \beta_0 + \beta_1 CPIC_t + \beta_2 U_t + \beta_3 Q_2 + \beta_4 Q_3 \\
& + \beta_5 Q_4
\end{aligned}
\tag{3.7}
$$

The system may be solved for total effects as before. As specified, equations 3.6 and 3.7 imply that the full effects of changes in explanatory variables are realized within one quarter. According to this specification, short-run and long-run effects are equal. Although the static model is perhaps less plausible, at least the Durbin-Watson (D-W) statistics obtained from the static regressions are reliable indicators of autocorrelation. With autocorrelation, the parameter estimate of the lagged dependent variable is biased and inconsistent. Moreover, with a lagged dependent variable included, the D-W statistic is misleading. One may gauge the degree of autocorrelation in our time series from the static regressions.[9]

Estimation of the Model

In order to estimate our model we used quarterly time-series data for the entire United States for the years 1969 through 1975, a total of twenty-eight observations. Definitions and descriptions of data sources are outlined in table 3-6.[10] All of the equations in our model are specified as linear. Underlying our specification is the assumption that our two-equation system is diagonally recursive. By this we mean that the health status variables that serve as explanatory factors in the utilization regression are not correlated with the utilization regression's disturbance. If the system is diagonally recursive, the application of ordinary least squares (OLS) to each of the two equations leads to consistent and asymptotically efficient parameter estimates.[11]

Empirical Results

The utilization regression results for all age categories combined are presented in table 3-7. Judging from the R^2s, the regressions explain more than 80 percent of the variation in utilization. The Durbin-Watson (D-W) statistics are around 2.0, suggesting that the residuals are not serially correlated.

Gauged in terms of statistical significance, the health status measures, restricted-activity days (RAD), and bed-disability days (BDD) dominate these regressions. The RAD coefficients suggest that a single restricted activity day generates one-tenth of a visit. By inference, at the margin, nine-tenths of restricted activity days do not involve visits to physicians. Not surprisingly, since confinement to bed represents more serious illness on the average, the BDD coefficients imply a somewhat higher visit response to bed disability; the coefficients range from 0.16 to 0.18 versus 0.11 to 0.12 for restricted activity days. The marginal impacts of RAD and BDD on visits should be distinguished from the average relationships, visits per restricted-activity and per bed-disability day, discussed earlier. Visits per unit of RAD and BDD are much higher than the marginal impacts implied by Table 3-7. The reason that the average impact exceeds the marginal impact is straightforward. Visits occur for many other reasons than for poor health on a given day. The average rates reflect this more strongly than do the marginal impacts. The regression coefficients indicate the increase in visits to be expected if restricted-activity and/or bed-disability days increased; the average rates can be very misleading on this count.

The inflation (CPIC) coefficients provide *some* evidence that, holding health status and other factors constant, an increase in the inflation rate lowers physicians' services utilization. However, the associated elasticities are very low (from −0.02 to −0.03). As noted in chapter 1, it is not possible to predict the effect of inflation on consumption on the basis of economic theory alone, and we gave reasons for the effect to be positive as well as negative. Table 3-7's results imply that the impact of inflation on physicians' services utilization is negative, on balance, but not very strongly so.

It is also impossible to predict the effect of unemployment on use a priori. The signs of the coefficients associated with the unemployment variable (U) are positive, but the U coefficients, unlike those for CPIC, never attain statistical significance. The positive signs provide weak evidence that the reductions in the time price resulting from unemployment dominate transitory income effects, which would reduce utilization. The utilization-unemployment elasticity is 0.12 at its highest (based on the U coefficient in regression 4). The impacts of unemployment on health insurance coverage and/or health status are approximated in the regressions by the variables REXP, RAD, and BDD. Therefore the forces underlying U's parameter estimates are largely confined to ("pure") income (of unemployed persons) and time-price effects and, consequently, understate the total effect of unemployment on utilization.

Real personal per capita income (YRP) measures the prosperity of families not directly affected by job loss as well as the unemployed. Our YRP series begins to fall in the fourth quarter of 1973. Even then, YRP was 4.1 percent below its peak reached in the third quarter of 1973. The decline in YRP actually preceded the worst periods of inflation and unemployment.

The significance of the YRP parameters depends to a considerable extent on whether the unemployment variable is included or not. Excluding U, YRP is statistically significant at conventional levels, or nearly so. The associated elasticities are high, from 0.42 to 1.26, higher than most "pure" income elasticities reported in past research with cross-sectional data.[12] The income variables in many of these studies refer to permanent income, and it is possible that transitory-cyclical fluctuations in personal income affect the timing of visits to the doctor. If so, time-series elasticity estimates may be relatively high.

Although the patient care physician-population ratio (MDSP) parameter estimates are positive, as anticipated, the estimates tend to be quite imprecise. Associated elasticities range from 0.31 to 1.09. We expected the percentage of expenditures on physicians' services covered by private and public third parties to have a positive impact on utilization, but the REXP parameter estimates are uniformly negative and statistically insignificant. Multicollinearity is possibly to blame in part; the simple correlation between REXP and MDSP is 0.94. With the exception of one minor downturn, the percentage of expenditures reimbursed rose monotonically over time, from 54.2 at the beginning to 61.2 percent at the end of the period included in our analysis. Public insurance clearly made up for losses in private coverage.

The lagged dependent variables' coefficients are 0.17 and 0.18 for regressions with RAD as the dependent variable and 0.24 and 0.28 for those based on BDD. Referring to equation 3.4, the fraction of the full impact of a change in an

Table 3-6
Variable Means, Definitions, and Sources: Time Series Analysis

Variable	Mean	Description	Source
BDDA	1.21	Days of bed disability, per person, for persons under 6 years.	Data are from the Health Interview Survey and are published in *Current Estimates, Vital and Health Statistics Series 10*, 1969–1975, U.S. Department of Health, Education, and Welfare, National Center for Health Statistics.
BDDB	1.08	Days of bed disability, per person, for persons 6–16 years.	See *BDDA* source.
BDDC	1.28	Days of bed disability, per person, for persons 17–44 years.	See *BDDA* source.
BDDD	1.93	Days of bed disability, per person, for persons 45–64 years.	See *BDDA* source.
BDDE	3.36	Days of bed disability, per person, for persons 65 years and older.	See *BDDA* source.
BDDT	1.57	Days of bed disability, per person, for all ages of the population.	See *BDDA* source.
CPIC	1.58	Quarterly rate of change in Consumer Price Index for all commodities (1969 = 100).	For the period 1969–1974 data are from *Business Statistics*, U.S. Department of Commerce. For 1975, data are from *Survey of Current Business*, U.S. Department of Commerce.
DVPA	1.54	Number of doctor visits, per person, for persons under 6 years.	Data are unpublished data from the Health Interview Survey.
DVPB	0.76	Number of doctor visits, per person, for persons 6–16 years.	See *DVPA* source.
DVPC	1.19	Number of doctor visits, per person, for persons 17–44 years.	See *DVPA* source.
DVPD	1.30	Number of doctor visits, per person, for persons 45–64 years.	See *DVPA* source.
DVPE	1.64	Number of doctor visits, per person, for persons 65 years and older.	See *DVPA* source.
DVPT	1.21	Number of doctor visits, per person, for all ages of the population.	See *DVPA* source.
MDSP[a]	0.0013	Number of nonfederal patient-care physicians per capita.	Physician data are from *Health Resources Statistics, 1975*, NCHS. Population are from *Business Statistics and Survey of Current Business*, U.S. Department of Commerce.

RADA	2.89	Days of restricted activity, per person, for persons under 6 years.	Data are from the Health Interview Survey and are published in Current Estimates, Vital and Health Statistics, Series 10, 1969–1975.
RADB	2.44	Days of restricted activity, per person, for persons 6–16 years.	See RADA source.
RADC	3.23	Days of restricted activity, per person, for persons 17–44 years.	See RADA source.
RADD	5.48	Days of restricted activity, per person, for persons 45–64 years.	See RADA source.
RADE	8.70	Days of restricted activity, per person, for persons 65 years and older	See RADA source.
RADT	4.02	Days of restricted activity, per person, for all ages of the population.	See RADA source.
REXP[a]	58.2	Proportion of expenditures for physician services that was met by third parties—government, private health insurance, philanthropy, and industry.	Data are from Social Security Bulletin, Social Security Administration.
U	5.66	Unemployment rate.	Data are from Business Statistics and Survey of Current Business. See U source.
YRP	3639.2	Real per capita income.	

[a]Quarterly data were not available, so we computed moving-average estimates of quarterly data. Our algorithm for constructing moving averages was:

$$X_{Q=\text{I}} = .6(X_t) + .4(X_{t-1}); \quad X_{Q=\text{II}} = .8(X_t) + .2(X_{t-1}); \quad X_{Q=\text{III}} = .8(X_t) + .2(X_{t+1}); \quad X_{Q=\text{IV}} = .6(X_t) + .4(X_{t+1})$$

where Q = quarter, t = current year. All other data are available on a quarterly (or monthly) basis.

Table 3-7
Utilization Regressions: All Age Categories Combined

Regression Number	Explanatory Variables									R^2 $R^2(C)$	D-W§
	CONS	YRP	MDSP	REXP	RAD	BDD	CPIC	U	L.DEP.		
1	0.14 (0.55)	0.00027 (0.00015)‡	488.2 (619.7)	-0.018 (0.019)	0.113 (0.016)*	— (–)	0.018 (0.018)	0.009 (0.016)	— (–)	0.85 0.80	2.11 –
2	-0.11 (0.32)	0.00020 (0.00009)†	566.2 (594.8)	-0.010 (0.013)	0.114 (0.015)*	— (–)	-0.026 (0.011)†	— (–)	— (–)	0.84 0.81	2.04 –
3	-0.06 (0.58)	0.00042 (0.00017)†	782.4 (655.8)	-0.028 (0.020)	— (–)	0.162 (0.025)*	0.012 (0.019)	0.025 (0.017)	— (–)	0.83 0.77	2.08 –
4	-0.78 (0.34)†	0.00023 (0.00010)†	1014.5 (656.3)	-0.006 (0.015)	— (–)	0.163 (0.026)*	-0.036 (0.012)*	— (–)	— (–)	0.81 0.76	1.88 –
5	0.16 (0.54)	0.00018 (0.00017)	292.6 (625.1)	-0.011 (0.019)	0.120 (0.017)*	— (–)	-0.018 (0.018)	0.004 (0.016)	0.168 (0.125)	0.86 0.81	–
6	0.07 (0.34)	0.00015 (0.00010)	312.9 (603.5)	-0.008 (0.013)	0.121 (0.016)*	— (–)	-0.021 (0.011)‡	— (–)	0.175 (0.118)	0.86 0.82	–
7	-0.05 (0.55)	0.00029 (0.00017)‡	524.9 (634.8)	-0.020 (0.020)	— (–)	0.181 (0.026)*	-0.013 (0.018)	0.018 (0.016)	0.244 (0.132)‡	0.85 0.80	–
8	-0.55 (0.33)	0.00014 (0.00010)	650.6 (629.6)	-0.003 (0.014)	— (–)	0.184 (0.026)*	-0.029 (0.013)†	— (–)	0.278 (0.130)†	0.84 0.80	–

*Significant at the 1 percent level; †Significant at the 5 percent level; ‡Significant at the 10 percent level; §Durbin-Watson statistic not applicable with lagged dependent variable.

independent variable realized within the first quarter is $1 - \alpha_7$, where α_7 is the parameter of the lagged dependent variable. It follows that 0.83 and 0.82 of the full response to changes in the explanatory variables is realized within the first quarter in the regressions using *RAD*. For those based on *BDD*, the comparable fractions are 0.76 and 0.72. These results imply that most of the response occurs quickly, and the short-run and long-run responses are thus not very different. In fact, the results imply that static models which exclude the lagged dependent variable also represent reasonable specifications. As noted above, the static specification assumes that the full response occurs within the quarter.

The regression results for the five age categories are presented in table 3-8. When compared to those in table 3-7, the R^2s are low, especially for the upper age groups. Moreover, the Durbin-Watson statistics suggest negative auto-correlation. With negative autocorrelation, parameter estimates of the lagged dependent variable have a negative bias. Although methods exist for obtaining consistent coefficients, we have not attempted to estimate the model in its dynamic form using such techniques for two reasons. First, the small sample size does not allow one to realize the advantages of consistency. Second, evidence from table 3-7 suggests that the static model provides a fairly good approximation of the underlying structure.

Table 3-8 displays a considerable amount of variation across age categories. Variation per se is not surprising. Restricted activity and bed disability days have different meanings at different ages. For young children, they are likely to be caused by acute illnesses. In older age groups, they are more likely to reflect chronic conditions. Other parameters are likely to vary because the aggregate measures of economic conditions have different impacts on individual age categories. Persons over age 65, for instance, may be less affected by unemployment, but could be more sensitive to high rates of inflation.

The utilization response to the two health status measures does indeed differ according to age. The coefficients are highest for the under 6 age group (*DVPA*) and lower for the age 6 to 16 (*DVPB*) and over age 65 (*DVPE*) categories. Because the two need measures have different meanings at different ages, one should not draw conclusions about age-dependent variations in access from table 3-8. However, such relationships cannot be ruled out on the basis of the results outlined in the table either. The unemployment parameters are, if anything, less reliable in table 3-8 than in table 3-7, but the inflation and real per capita income effects are sometimes larger than in the preceding table.

Health status regressions are contained in table 3-9. The variables Q_2, Q_3, and Q_4 adjust for seasonality. The fact that these variables uniformly have a statistically significant impact on restricted-activity and bed-disability days is an indication that both variables partly reflect acute illnesses, which are most likely to occur during the first three months of the year.

More interesting from a public policy perspective are the impacts of unemployment and inflation on the two health status measures. Unemployment has

Table 3-8
Utilization Regressions by Age Category

Regression Number	Dependent Variable	CONS	YRP	MDSP	Explanatory Variables REXP	RAD	BDD	CPIC	U	R^2 $R^2(C)$	D-W
1	DVPA	-1.81 (1.35)	0.00096 (0.00379)	2139.2 (1503.)	-0.0002 (0.0477)	0.173 (0.022)*	– (–)	-0.0828 (0.0441)‡	-0.019 (0.039)	0.81 0.76	2.54 –
2	DVPA	-1.27 (0.75)	0.00024 (0.00023)	1975.4 (1439.)	-0.0172 (0.0319)	0.171 (0.021)*	– (–)	-0.0655 (0.0257)†	– (–)	0.81 0.76	2.55 –
3	DVPA	-2.62 (1.62)	-0.00005 (0.00045)	1657.7 (1776.)	0.0359 (0.0580)	– (–)	0.362 (0.059)*	-0.1108 (0.0530)†	-0.027 (0.047)	0.74 0.66	2.36 –
4	DVPA	-1.85 (0.89)†	0.00016 (0.00027)	1446.3 (1709.)	0.011 (0.0381)	– (–)	0.353 (0.056)	-0.0860 (0.0304)*	– (–)	0.73 0.67	2.39 –
5	DVPB	0.36 (0.73)	0.00013 (0.00021)	-30.8 (820.6)	-0.0040 (0.0262)	0.041 (0.013)*	– (–)	0.0114 (0.0240)	0.014 (0.021)	0.53 0.39	2.76 –
6	DVPB	-0.02 (0.41)	0.00003 (0.00012)	79.3 (791.5)	0.0084 (0.0175)	0.043 (0.012)*	– (–)	-0.0011 (0.0140)	– (–)	0.52 0.41	2.62 –
7	DVPB	0.46 (0.72)	0.00018 (0.00020)	-89.9 (808.2)	-0.0078 (0.0251)	– (–)	0.068 (0.020)*	0.0157 (0.0234)	0.020 (0.021)	0.55 0.41	2.67 –
8	DVPB	-0.12 (0.41)	0.00002 (0.00012)	85.4 (788.5)	0.0106 (0.0176)	– (–)	0.070 (0.020)*	-0.0029 (0.0190)	– (–)	0.53 0.41	2.44 –
9	DVPC	0.00 (1.03)	0.00028 (0.00029)	147.1 (1163.)	-0.0070 (0.0362)	0.135 (0.036)*	– (–)	-0.0188 (0.0337)	0.000 (0.030)	0.61 0.50	2.43 –
10	DVPC	-0.00 (0.59)	0.00027 (0.00017)	148.4 (1102.)	-0.0069 (0.0248)	0.135 (0.035)*	– (–)	-0.0188 (0.0198)	– (–)	0.61 0.52	2.43 –
11	DVPC	-0.27 (1.02)	0.00036 (0.00028)	345.5 (1145.)	-0.0090 (0.0356)	– (–)	0.203 (0.052)*	-0.0236 (0.0321)	0.006 (0.029)	0.63 0.52	2.51 –
12	DVPC	-0.43 (0.57)	0.00031 (0.00017)‡	399.3 (1085.)	-0.0042 (0.0243)	– (–)	0.204 (0.051)*	-0.0288 (0.0194)	– (–)	0.62 0.54	2.49 –

13	DVPD	-0.15 (3.28)	0.00130 (0.00089)	2162.9 (3649.)	-0.1268 (0.1144)	0.144 (0.088)	— (—)	0.0034 (0.1057)	0.094 (0.093)	0.40 0.23	2.35 —
14	DVPD	-2.84 (1.95)	0.00059 (0.00056)	3028.3 (3551.)	-0.0442 (0.0804)	0.147 (0.088)	— (—)	-0.0819 (0.0643)	— (—)	0.37 0.22	2.28 —
15	DVPD	-0.92 (3.30)	0.00139 (0.00091)	2520.2 (3713.)	-0.1200 (0.1162)	— (—)	0.185 (0.135)	-0.0112 (0.1074)	0.098 (0.095)	0.38 0.20	2.38 —
16	DVPD	-3.74 (1.89)	0.00065 (0.00057)	3429.0 (3615.)	-0.0336 (0.0812)	— (—)	0.187 (0.135)	-0.1004 (0.0647)	— (—)	0.35 0.19	2.29 —
17	DVPE	1.84 (1.01)‡	0.00043 (0.00027)	-869.7 (1127.)	-0.0244 (0.0344)	0.073 (0.026)*	— (—)	0.0061 (0.0319)	0.023 (0.028)	0.47 0.31	2.71 —
18	DVPE	1.18 (0.61)	0.00026 (0.00017)	-654.0 (1088.)	-0.0041 (0.0239)	0.073 (0.025)*	— (—)	-0.0149 (0.0193)	— (—)	0.45 0.35	2.77 —
19	DVPE	1.04 (1.11)	0.00038 (0.00031)	26.0 (1248.)	-0.0189 (0.0392)	— (—)	0.048 (0.036)	-0.0009 (0.0036)	0.026 (0.032)	0.31 0.10	2.18 —
20	DVPE	0.30 (0.64)	0.00018 (0.00019)	258.7 (1206.)	0.0044 (0.0269)	— (—)	0.045 (0.035)	-0.0247 (0.0215)	— (—)	0.29 0.16	2.28 —

*Significant at the 1 percent level; †Significant at the 5 percent level; ‡Significant at the 10 percent level.

Table 3-9
Health Status Regressions

Regression Number	Dependent Variable	Explanatory Variables						R^2	$R^2(C)$	D-W
		CONS	Q_2	Q_3	Q_4	CPIC	U			
1	RADT	3.65 (0.17)*	-0.98 (0.098)*	-1.26 (0.098)*	-0.71 (0.098)*	0.171 (0.039)*	0.152 (0.024)*	0.92	0.90	0.65
2	RADA	3.32 (0.28)*	-1.48 (0.166)*	-1.88 (0.164)*	-0.30 (0.163)‡	0.069 (0.065)	0.074 (0.040)‡	0.90	0.88	2.55
3	RADB	3.23 (0.27)*	-1.62 (0.124)*	-2.06 (0.124)*	-1.16 (0.124)*	0.091 (0.050)‡	0.057 (0.030)‡	0.91	0.92	2.16
4	RADC	2.93 (0.19)*	-0.92 (0.108)*	-0.87 (0.108)*	-0.41 (0.108)*	0.127 (0.043)*	0.119 (0.026)*	0.86	0.83	1.42
5	RADD	4.64 (0.34)*	-0.71 (0.197)*	-1.18 (0.197)*	-0.74 (0.196)*	0.213 (0.078)*	0.217 (0.048)*	0.77	0.71	1.36
6	RADE	6.64 (0.52)*	-0.20 (0.306)	-0.56 (0.306)‡	-0.68 (0.306)†	0.290 (0.122)†	0.350 (0.075)*	0.62	0.52	1.24
7	BDDT	1.93 (0.08)*	-0.69 (0.044)*	-0.82 (0.044)*	-0.49 (0.044)*	0.050 (0.018)*	0.014 (0.011)	0.95	0.94	1.65
8	BDDA	1.70 (0.14)*	-0.74 (0.082)*	-0.86 (0.082)*	-0.21 (0.082)*	0.029 (0.033)	-0.010 (0.020)	0.88	0.85	2.31
9	BDDB	1.89 (0.11)*	-1.07 (0.065)*	-1.27 (0.065)*	-0.77 (0.065)*	0.032 (0.026)	-0.010 (0.016)	0.95	0.94	2.13
10	BDDC	1.40 (0.89)*	-0.59 (0.052)*	-0.65 (0.052)*	-0.32 (0.052)*	0.058 (0.021)*	0.033 (0.013)*	0.91	0.89	1.99
11	BDDD	2.03 (0.15)*	-0.62 (0.087)*	-0.83 (0.087)*	-0.59 (0.087)*	0.076 (0.035)†	0.054 (0.021)†	0.84	0.80	1.68
12	BDDE	3.91 (0.32)*	-0.71 (0.189)*	-0.75 (0.189)*	-0.48 (0.189)†	-0.024 (0.075)	-0.000 (0.046)	0.48	0.36	1.93

*Significant at the 1 percent level; †Significant at the 5 percent level; ‡Significant at the 10 percent level.

a statistically significant, positive impact on health status in the total (*RADT* and *BDDT*) and prime working-age adult regressions (*RADC, RADD, BDDC, BDDD*). Unemployment coefficients for the other age groups tend to be less significant, and in some cases, even negative. These results imply that job loss affects the health of the "at-risk" group, the adult prime working age. With one exception (the *BDDE* regression), the inflation (*CPIC*) parameter estimates are also positive, and at least for the prime working age groups, they tend to be statistically significant. Not surprisingly, the impacts of unemployment and inflation are larger in the restricted-activity than in the bed-disability day regressions. On the whole, the results displayed in table 3-9 confirm Brenner's finding that adverse economic conditions result in lower health status.[13]

Table 3-10 contains reduced form utilization equations for both static and dynamic variants of the model. The reduced form gives the total effects of the two-equation model's exogenous variables on utilization. As noted previously, the total effect is the sum of both the direct effect of exogenous variables on utilization shown in tables 3-7 and 3-8 and the indirect effects of exogenous variables affecting utilization via their effect on health status.

Since, as reflected in table 3-9, inflation tends to increase restricted activity and bed disability days which in turn raise utilization; the health effect of inflation partly or fully offsets the generally negative direct effect of inflation on utilization. Hence, the total effect of inflation on utilization tends to be very small. Utilization-inflation elasticities, based on the reduced form coefficients from equations 3.1 through 3.4 in table 3-10, are zero.

The effect of unemployment on health status tends to be positive; therefore, when the direct effect of unemployment is also positive (which is most often the case), the two effects reinforce one another. For example, the 0.025 parameter in table 3-7 (regression number 3) rises to 0.027 when the indirect effect is also considered. Thus, the highest utilization-unemployment elasticity associated with the "total" regressions reported in table 3-10 is 0.15 (versus 0.14 in table 3-7). This elasticity gives the utilization response within the first quarter. The corresponding long-run elasticity is 0.20. Comparing the *total effects* of unemployment and inflation, unemployment has a more pronounced impact on the use of physicians' services on the average.

Summary and Conclusions

In this chapter we have presented both cross-tabular and regression analyses of unpublished data from the Health Interview Surveys for the years 1969-1975. Our cross-tabulations assess annual means, often disaggregated on the basis of age, income, family size, and employment status. The regressions are based on a time series of quarterly observations covering the same period. There are two types of dependent variables: visits to physicians and health status measures.

Table 3-10
Reduced Form Utilization Equations

Equation Number	Dependent Variable	Based on Table Numbers	Regression Numbers	Explanatory Variables									
				CONS	YRP	MDSP	REXP	CPIC	U	Q_2	Q_3	Q_4	L. DEP
1	$DVPT_{RADT}$	20, 22	1, 1	0.54	0.00027	488.2	-0.018	0.001	0.026	-0.11	-0.14	-0.08	—
2	$DVPT_{BDDT}$	20, 22	3, 7	0.60	0.00042	782.4	-0.028	0.003	0.027	-0.12	-0.15	-0.09	0.17
3	$DVPT_{RADT}$	20, 22	5, 1	0.25	0.00018	292.6	-0.011	-0.004	0.027	-0.11	-0.13	-0.08	—
4	$DVPT_{BDDT}$	20, 22	7, 7	0.30	0.00029	524.9	-0.020	-0.004	0.021	-0.14	-0.15	-0.09	0.24
5	$DVPA_{RADA}$	21, 21	1, 2	-1.24	0.00095	2139.2	-0.0002	-0.071	-0.006	-0.26	-0.33	-0.05	—
6	$DVPA_{BDDA}$	21, 22	3, 8	-2.00	-0.00005	1656.7	-0.36	-0.101	-0.031	-0.27	-0.31	-0.08	—
7	$DVPB_{RADB}$	21, 22	5, 3	0.49	0.00013	-30.8	-0.004	0.015	0.016	-0.07	-0.09	-0.05	—
8	$DVPB_{BDDB}$	21, 22	7, 9	0.44	0.00018	-89.9	-0.008	0.012	0.011	-0.04	-0.05	-0.03	—
9	$DVPC_{RADC}$	21, 22	9, 4	0.40	0.00028	147.1	-0.007	-0.002	0.016	-0.12	-0.12	-0.06	—
10	$DVPC_{BDDC}$	21, 22	11, 10	-0.08	0.00036	345.5	-0.009	-0.016	0.010	-0.08	-0.09	-0.04	—
11	$DVPD_{RADD}$	21, 22	13, 5	0.52	0.00130	2162.9	-0.127	0.034	0.037	-0.10	-0.17	-0.11	—
12	$DVPD_{BDDD}$	21, 22	15, 11	-0.54	0.00139	2520.2	-0.120	0.003	0.108	-0.11	-0.15	-0.11	—
13	$DVPE_{RADE}$	21, 22	17, 6	2.32	0.00043	-869.7	-0.024	0.027	0.049	-0.01	-0.04	-0.05	—
14	$DVPE_{BDDE}$	21, 22	19, 12	1.23	0.00038	26.0	-0.019	-0.002	0.03	-0.03	-0.04	-0.02	—

Since the same health status variables appear as explanatory variables in the visits regressions, we are able to assess the indirect effects of inflation and unemployment on utilization of physicians' services as well as the direct effects. We were led to the notion that adverse economic conditions may affect health by the pioneering work of Brenner.

There are several principal results of our cross-tabular analysis. First, there was a secular upward trend in visits per capita over the 1969-1975 period. However, when one divides the visits series by a measure of health status—restricted-activity days or, alternatively, bed-disability days—this trend disappears. Specific effects of the 1974-1975 inflation-recession cannot be discerned from these cross-tabulations.

Second, there is substantial variation in visit rates by demographic group. Furthermore, differences in growth in visits per capita over the 1969-1975 period are evident by demographic group. Visit rates for the under age 17 category grew comparatively fast; by contrast, growth of visits for the post-age 65 group grew relatively slowly. These differential growth rates are understandable when one considers that Medicare has covered physicians' services for the vast majority of elderly persons since 1966.

Third, tabulations clearly show that persons living in lower income households tend to be in poorer health.

Fourth, the proportion of total physicians' visits occurring in hospital outpatient departments and emergency rooms increased over 1974-1975 while the proportion of home visits declined. We offer several explanations for these developments. Among these is the inflation-recession of 1974-1975. Although the marked increases in outpatient department and emergency room visit proportions during 1974-1975 would seem to suggest that inflation-recession is indeed a reason for increased patient use of physicians at these sites, there is also some contrary evidence. In particular, while the poor consistently depend on these sources of care more than others, there is no evidence that the poor's dependence on these sources increased comparatively rapidly during 1974-1975. Certainly the effects of recessions tend to be borne disproportionately by the poor. Choice of site of care is the subject of much more in-depth investigation in chapter 5.

Finally, persons unemployed at the time of the survey report 34 percent more visits per capita than the employed. However, when visits are expressed in terms of our two health status measures, the currently unemployed appear to have much lower levels of access to ambulatory care. The unemployed clearly have poorer health on the average. This association *suggests* that job loss causes a loss in health status; however, one must be cautious about such a conclusion since it is also possible that causation runs in the opposite direction—from health to employment status. The latter type of causation is much less likely to be dominant in an aggregate quarterly time-series than in a cross-section.[14]

There are several important results from the regression analysis. First, real per capita income exerts a strong positive impact on the utilization of physicians' services. Our elasticity estimates are in the 0.4 to 1.3 range. These are larger on the whole than income elasticities obtained by others in cross-sectional analysis. The difference may be largely attributed to the postponable nature of many kinds of physicians' services. The tendency to defer visits to physicians in the short run and intermediate run is relatively easy to detect with a quarterly time-series.

Second, the regressions suggest that the inflation rate has a negative direct effect on utilization. This negative impact is in large part attributable to the hedging phenomenon described in chapter 1. However, the inflation rate also demonstrates a positive effect on our two health status measures, restricted-activity days and bed-disability days. These variables in turn have positive impacts on visits to physicians. The indirect effect of inflation operating through health status almost entirely offsets its direct effect. Thus, the total effect of inflation on visits to physicians is essentially nil. Inflation's effects are best assessed with a time series. This is the major result on inflation's impact in this study.

Third, the direct effect of unemployment on utilization is less clearly evident from our visit regressions than is that of inflation. Positive coefficients are consistently obtained on our unemployment variable, implying the dominance of time-price effects over forces associated with unemployment that tend to diminish use. We find that unemployment raises the number of restricted and disability days. Unlike inflation, the indirect effect of unemployment operating via health status reinforces the positive direct effect. Thus, the total impact of increased unemployment on utilization of physicians' services is positive.

Fourth, we also assessed the effects of physician availability and the proportion of expenditures on physicians' services covered by both private and public third parties. Neither variable has a statistically significant impact on utilization. In part, poor results are attributable to the lack of cyclical or other short-term variation in either series. The insurance coverage proportion rose monotonically, with one minor exception, throughout the 1969–1975 period.

Finally, our results imply that about three-quarters of the complete effect on visits of a change in the level of an explanatory variable is realized in the quarter in which the change occurs. This is a quite rapid response.

Notes

1. Certainly these measures are far from ideal, but they are about the only health status-related measures available on an annual basis.

2. Although health status-adjusted visit series such as these are often used for making normative inferences, we have some reservations about this. First, as noted above, a hypochondriac may have many sick days, but are we to insist that he or she have a commensurately larger number of visits? Second, reasons

for visits vary markedly across population groups. Children, for example, receive a substantial amount of preventive care. Are we then to infer from health status-adjusted visits measures, such as those presented in table 3-3, that children have the best access to physician care?

3. Judith D. Bentkover and Claudia R. Saunders, *Trends in Facility Use: An Evaluation of the Impact of Adverse Economic Conditions on the Health Status of the Poor,* Final Report on Contract No. HRA 230-75-123, Policy Analysis, Inc., Brookline, Massachusetts, 1977.

4. To conserve space these tables are not presented here; they are available from the authors on request.

5. Inflation could, of course, also be seen as a supply variable.

6. M. Harvey Brenner, *Estimating Social Costs of National Economic Policy: Implications for Mental and Physical Health and Criminal Aggression,* Washington: Joint Economic Committee of the U.S. Congress, October 1976.

7. Victor Fuchs and Marcia Kramer, *Determinants of Expenditures for Physicians' Services in the United States, 1948–1968,* Washington: U.S. Department of Health, Education, and Welfare, National Center for Health Services Research, 1972.

8. For a more thorough discussion of this point, see Frank Sloan and Roger Feldman, "Competition Among Physicians," in Warren Greenberg (ed.), *Competition in the Health Care Sector: Past, Present, and Future,* Proceedings of a Conference Sponsored by the Federal Trade Commission, March 1978, pp. 57–131.

9. Assuming a partial equilibrium adjustment model, inclusion of a lagged dependent variable does not introduce autocorrelation. See Zvi Griliches, "Distributed Lags: A Survey," *Econometrica* 35:16–49, 1967. See J. Johnston, *Econometric Methods,* New York: McGraw-Hill, 1972, for a general discussion of this problem.

10. The time-series feature as well as the twenty-eight observations limit the number and types of variables that can be included.

11. Even if one were to quarrel with the assumption that the two-equation system is diagonally recursive, it is doubtful one would gain much by using a simultaneous equation technique, considering the small number of degrees of freedom.

12. See, for example, Ronald Andersen and Lee Benham, "Factors Affecting the Relationship Between Family Income and Medical Care Consumption," in H. Klarman (ed.), *Empirical Studies in Health Economics,* Baltimore: Johns Hopkins University Press, 1970, pp. 73–95; Lee Benham and Alexandra Benham, "Utilization of Physician Services Across Income Groups, 1963–1970," in Ronald Andersen, et al. (eds.) *Equity in Health Services,* Cambridge, Massachusetts: Ballinger Publishing Co., 1975, pp. 97–194; Joseph P. Newhouse and Charles E. Phelps, "New Estimates of Price and Income Elasticities of Medical Care Services," in Richard Rosett (ed.), *The Role of Health Insurance in the*

Health Services Sector, New York: National Bureau of Economic Research, 1976, pp. 261-312; Charles E. Phelps, "Effects of Insurance on Demand for Medical Care," in Ronald Andersen, et al. (eds.), *Equity in Health Services,* Cambridge, Massachusetts: Ballinger Publishing Co., 1975, pp. 105-130.

13. Brenner, *Estimating Social Costs.*

14. For a discussion of the effects of health status on employment and earnings, see Harold S. Luft, "The Impact of Poor Health on Earnings," *Review of Economics and Statistics* 57 (February 1975):43-57.

4

Access in 1974:
A Cross-Sectional
Analysis

In Chapter 3, we presented a fairly detailed analysis of the utilization dimension of the access to medical care. In this chapter, we broaden the scope of our inquiry to assess process and satisfaction dimensions of access. In particular, we investigate the descriptors of qualitative and convenience aspects of the patient's contact with the health care system. As in chapter 3, we use both cross-tabular and multivariate analyses to draw inferences concerning the effects of adverse economic conditions on access.

The empirical evidence for this chapter pertains to 1974. Although unemployment was not as high in 1974 as in 1975, it began to increase substantially, especially by the fall. Inflation was at its highest level in recent history. Prices rose at double-digit rates all year. Real per capita income had begun to decline in 1973 and continued to do so throughout 1974.

Data for this chapter come from the 1974 Health Interview Survey (HIS). The HIS covers a sample of civilian, noninstitutionalized persons and includes measures of perceived health status and access to medical care. Although the HIS has been conducted on a regular basis since 1957, the 1974 survey included a special section focusing on several process and satisfaction dimensions of access to medical care. The process measures concern the presence and type of usual source of ambulatory care as well as the presence and type of problems encountered in obtaining care. The satisfaction measures reflect perceptions of the amount of care received versus the amount of care needed. Our research in this chapter is based on our own empirical analysis of public use of tapes made available by the National Center for Health Statistics (NCHS).

Three basic questions are addressed in this chapter. First, given that the economy deteriorated rapidly during 1974, was this economy-wide decline reflected in a decrease in Americans' access to ambulatory care? Second, as of 1974, how did the employed and unemployed compare along several dimensions of access? Third, how did the access of the short-term and the long-term unemployed compare? The HIS data base is unique among data sources containing access information in allowing one to distinguish among the unemployed according to the duration of unemployment.[1]

Cross-Tabular Investigation

Table 4--1 contains responses by household heads to HIS questions on process and satisfaction dimensions of access, respectively, As defined in chapter 1,

Table 4-1
Process and Satisfaction Indexes of Access

Index	Entire Sample			Percentage of Household Heads Aged 25-64			
		Quarter		Income Below $7,000		Income $7,000 and Higher	
	Annual	First	Fourth	Employed	Unemployed	Employed	Unemployed
Process							
Have usual source of care (particular MD or place)	80.4	81.0	79.7	86.4	84.6	87.3	84.9
Place of usual care							
Private doctor's office	61.3	60.7	61.0	66.3	41.7	70.1	67.8
Doctor's clinic	9.0	10.1	8.8	10.3	23.5	10.3	7.0
Group practice	1.9	1.5	2.4	0.7	7.5	2.2	4.5
Hospital outpatient clinic	3.8	3.5	3.8	3.4	0.0	2.4	2.8
Hospital emergency room	0.4	0.5	0.3	1.1	4.4	0.2	0.6
Other, unknown	4.0	4.7	3.4	4.4	7.5	2.1	2.2
Any problems getting medical care in last 12 months	10.4	10.8	10.4	13.8	15.4	12.4	19.0
Specific problems in getting care during last 12 months							
No doctor available when needed	2.7	2.9	2.8	3.9	7.8	3.1	4.6
No doctor available delayed care	2.2	2.2	2.4	3.4	7.8	2.2	3.0
No doctor available prevented care	0.7	0.9	0.7	2.0	3.9	0.9	1.5
Cost	2.6	2.6	2.7	6.0	7.9	1.4	6.2
Cost delayed care	2.0	2.1	2.2	4.5	7.9	1.2	5.2
Cost prevented care	1.5	1.6	1.5	4.2	7.9	0.8	3.1
Lack of Transportation	1.2	1.4	1.2	0.4	3.6	0.2	0.5
Lack of transportation delayed care	0.9	1.0	0.8	0.4	3.6	0.2	0.5
Lack of transportation prevented care	0.4	0.5	0.4	0.4	3.6	0.1	0.5
Inconvenient office hours	1.7	1.8	1.7	0.4	0.0	2.3	2.6
Inconvenient office hours delayed care	1.2	1.2	1.1	0.0	0.0	1.6	2.1
Inconvenient office hours prevented care	0.4	0.4	0.4	0.4	0.0	0.6	1.5
Problem getting appointment	5.0	4.9	5.1	5.4	7.8	7.8	11.3
Problem getting appointment delayed care	3.6	3.3	3.8	3.8	7.8	5.7	8.0
Problem getting appointment prevented care	1.0	1.1	1.0	2.3	7.8	1.7	3.3

Sources of payment for doctor's bills (Source used during last 12 months)							
Self or family	59.5	60.3	59.5	70.4	57.7	75.8	77.5
Medicare	4.2	4.0	4.5	0.0	0.0	0.2	1.0
Health insurance	23.5	22.8	24.1	16.4	24.1	33.9	44.9
Workman's compensation	1.3	1.4	1.1	1.5	0.0	1.2	1.7
Accident insurance (carried by family or person outside family)	1.0	1.2	1.1	0.9	5.5	0.7	1.5
Medicaid	2.5	2.3	2.7	0.7	7.5	0.1	0.5
Welfare	3.2	3.0	3.2	3.6	12.7	0.2	2.0
Satisfaction							
Persons receiving as much care as needed	89.7	90.3	89.2	86.1	88.6	92.4	86.4
Persons not receiving as much care as needed	6.0	6.4	5.8	12.5	11.4	5.0	10.3
Unknown whether there are unmet needs	4.4	3.3	5.0	1.5	0.0	2.6	3.3
Reasons for not receiving enough care							
Health care is too expensive	2.9	3.1	2.8	9.2	7.9	1.9	5.6
Difficulty getting to doctor	0.5	0.6	0.4	0.5	0.0	0.1	0.0
Can't get appointments	0.8	0.9	0.8	1.9	3.5	0.8	2.1
Office hours inconvenient	0.4	0.4	0.3	0.8	0.0	0.5	0.5
Doctor spends inadequate time	0.8	0.9	0.8	0.8	0.0	1.0	1.6

Source: National Center in Health Statistics 1974, Health Interview Survey (unpublished data).

process indexes describe the qualitative aspects of the patient's contact with the health care system. Satisfaction measures of access describe individuals' feelings about the medical care they or others receive.

It is generally recognized that persons with usual sources of care have better continuity of care. Aday and Anderson[2] found that people who have a usual physician are more apt to be satisfied with the care they receive than others who do not visit a usual provider. Other studies have related usual source to ambulatory care use,[3] but such links are somewhat suspect since it is difficult to assume one-way causation from usual source to use. Heavy users are more likely, holding other factors constant, to obtain a regular source.

Table 4-1 contains responses to a question regarding the usual source of ambulatory care. As in other surveys, the usual source question in the 1974 HIS refers to a particular physician or place. In terms of continuity of care, most experts maintain that it makes a considerable difference whether the patient has a usual physician or a usual place of care. In 1974, 80.4 percent of respondents had a usual source of care.[4] Of these, very few identified hospital outpatient clinics and emergency rooms as usual sources. While these settings have a function in the health care delivery system, they are not usually designed to provide "first line" care.

Interviewees were asked a very general "process" question: "During the past 12 months, have you had any problems getting medical care for—(for any of the following reasons)?" Among all respondents, 10.4 percent indicated that they had a problem among these listed by the interviewer. "Problem getting appointment" was mentioned by nearly half of the persons with a problem (5.0/10.4). "No doctor available" was the second most frequently listed problem. The HIS also determined whether a specific problem delayed and/or prevented the respondent from obtaining medical care. Responses to these questions are also reported in table 4-1.

As a general measure of satisfaction, the 1974 HIS asked whether or not people perceived they were receiving as much care as needed and, more specifically, the reported reasons for *not* receiving enough care. As seen in table 4-1, 89.7 percent of the sample felt that they "were receiving as much care as they needed." Reasons that the 6.0 percent of the respondents who stated that they had unmet needs given for their situation include the items listed at the bottom of table 4-1. Of these, "health care is too expensive" was mentioned most frequently.

This chapter's first objective is to compare responses to the HIS received in the first three months of 1974 with those obtained during the last three months in order to determine whether access to physicians' services deteriorated during the course of the year. Since his data were available to us on tapes, we were able to make quarterly comparisons on a number of access variables.

As table 4-1 shows, the changes from the first to the fourth quarter of 1974 were minimal, and not always in the same direction. For instance, a slightly smaller percentage of respondents stated that they had a usual source of care (81.0 versus 79.7 percent in the fourth quarter). But fewer persons stated that they had encountered problems obtaining medical care in the last twelve months (10.8 versus 10.4 percent in the fourth quarter) and explicitly stated that they had unmet needs at the time (6.4 versus 5.8 percent). There is some evidence from table 4-1 that the use of Medicaid increased during 1974, but the use of other third-party sources rose as well. More extensive tabulations, not reported here, support this conclusion based on table 4-1. In terms of table 4-1's measures, access to physicians' services remained essentially constant during 1974 for the U.S. population as a whole.

Table 4-1 also presents data for household heads by employment status (during the two weeks prior to the survey) and family income during the previous twelve months. The currently unemployed include household heads who during the prior two weeks:

Did not work, had a job, were on layoff;

Did not work, had a job, were on layoff and looking for work;

Did not work, had a job, but it is unknown if they were looking for work or on layoff;

Did not work, had no job, were looking for work or on layoff.[5]

The employed category is restricted to household heads who actually worked during the past two weeks. Household heads, not working but with a job and not on layoff, those not working but with a job and looking for another job, and those not in the labor force have been entirely excluded from the employed-unemployed comparisons. As constructed, the definitions of employment status in table 4-1 do not reveal anything about long-term employment.

The percentages reported in table 4-1 indicate that, regardless of income group, employed household heads were more likely than were unemployed heads to see one particular doctor, to be cared for at a private office or doctor's clinic, and to rely on employee benefits and Workmen's Compensation to cover medical expenses. Unemployed heads of a given age and income group were more likely to see more than one particular doctor, visit emergency rooms and clinics, use the telephone to communicate with the doctor, receive house calls, and rely on health insurance[6] and welfare for payment of medical bills. Furthermore, the unemployed experienced more severe problems in obtaining care. In particular, the unemployed more frequently encountered unavailability of a physician, "prohibitive" costs, lack of knowledge concerning the appropriate place to receive care, lack of transportation, inconvenient office hours, and difficulties in obtaining appointments. As a result of these barriers, the unemployed had, according to survey responses, a higher incidence of postponed and precluded care. The fact that the higher income unemployed were more likely to experience problems in obtaining care than the unemployed with lower incomes was unexpected.

Considering all employed household heads, those in the higher income group were more likely to have one particular doctor, receive treatment at a doctor's office or group practice, and either pay their own medical bills or have them covered by health insurance. Employed heads reporting income less than $7,000 were, on the other hand, more likely to receive treatment at a doctor's clinic or at a hospital outpatient or emergency room, and to rely on reimbursement by Workmen's Compensation or accident insurance carried by either a family member or a person outside of the family. Whereas heads in the higher income group cited inconvenient office hours and difficulties obtaining appointments as problems, lower income heads were more likely to report problems related to the cost of medical care.

A comparison between two income groups of the unemployed persons reflects the expected tendencies for higher income persons to receive treatment in a private office, and to use their own funds or private health insurance to pay bills. Lower income persons, by contrast, were treated in the clinic or emergency room, relied on Medicaid and welfare for payment of medical bills, and encountered cost and doctor availability problems.

Satisfaction with the level of care received is related to family income. For household heads in the over $7,000 income category, there are differences according to employment status. For heads with family income below $7,000, proportionately fewer unemployed reported unmet health care needs.

Although the percentages in table 4-1 generally support the view that the unemployed have lower access, the findings should be regarded as tentative for several reasons. First, many of the differences are small. The percentages with a usual source of care range from 84.6 to 87.3; percentages of heads with one or more problems obtaining medical care range from 12.4 to 19.0. Second, in some cases, there are unanticipated patterns. For instance, while the unemployed were more likely to report problems obtaining care than the employed, the high-income unemployed were more likely to have a problem than were unemployed heads with low incomes. Third, table 4-1 does not distinguish between short- and long-term unemployment. Fourth, while the table's frequency distributions present the HIS data in a relatively compact form and provide worthwhile insights, there is additional information which can be obtained from multivariate analysis. Regression analysis allows one to isolate the individual effects of a number of explanatory factors on access. It is used in the next section to analyze the impact of unemployment on the process and satisfaction dimensions of access.

Multivariate Investigation

In this section we first discuss general conceptual considerations. Then we present our empirical specification. Finally, we discuss our empirical results.

The three binary dependent variables to be analyzed are: (1) a variable which assumes the value one if the respondent had a usual source of care and is equal to zero otherwise; (2) a variable which equals one if the respondent encountered problems in obtaining medical care within the past twelve months and is equal to zero otherwise; and (3) a variable that takes the value one if the respondent felt that all his health care needs were met and zero otherwise. The regression analysis is limited to household heads age 25 and over.

Conceptual Considerations

To our knowledge, although they are often used, no previous study has developed a conceptual approach for analyzing these three access variables. It is therefore useful to begin with comments on their analytic content.

As noted above, a usual source of care is thought to provide patients with continuity of care. Private practitioners are most likely to provide continuity of care, although it is clear that not all of them do. Continuity of care is an "amenity" in the sense that this term was defined in chapter 2. And it is an amenity that the poor may well not be able to afford. Persons who lose their jobs may switch from private sector to hospital-based sources which require a lower out-of-pocket payment from the financially disadvantaged. The primary objective of the regression analysis of usual source is to determine whether family income and employment status affect the probability of possessing a usual source and, if there is a relationship, to determine how responsive the probability is to income and employment status.

The HIS listed a number of potential problems that respondents might have in obtaining ambulatory care. A head has been classified as having "any problems" if any item from the list was checked. The problems roughly fall into categories of out-of-pocket money prices, time prices, and availability-convenience. Prices, of course, are quite necessary "problems" because they serve to allocate scarce resources among alternative uses. Society has determined that a certain class of goods and services, called "merit wants," are not to be distributed according to the rule that price covers the marginal cost of production.[7] Medical care, which is heavily subsidized at the point of consumption, is a merit want. Nevertheless, some out-of-pocket payments for medical care are generally required. If one conducts a survey in which respondents are questioned about the burden of the price they pay for medical care, one should expect to find a pattern in the responses. In particular, lower income persons for whom medical care expenditures represent a higher proportion of their total budgets would be more likely to register complaints.

Time prices, by contrast, are likely to be a special burden to persons with high opportunity wages, often the affluent. However, given the way the HIS phrased the time price items, one cannot be certain that the affluent would be the most likely to complain about the time price. Low-income working persons may experience greater difficulties getting time off from work than persons in professional and managerial positions and therefore complain about "inconvenient office hours" and "problems getting an appointment."

Having "a doctor available when needed" is an amenity in the sense we use the term. Standby capacity is by no means costless. Resources, including physician time, are devoted to providing care when needed. Again, the financially disadvantaged may have less access to this amenity. Because they often lack an established relationship with a physician, the poor may experience greater difficulty obtaining nonemergent care immediately.

For years, economists have emphasized the distinction between need and demand, but, perhaps as testimony to their collective influence on the public, the need concept continues to find its way into policy discussions. In fact, in the medical care context, the term remains quite popular. Recognizing that the term is not likely to disappear, economists have attempted to give need a technical meaning. According to one definition, need is the amount that would be demanded at a zero out-of-pocket price to the patient. Unfortunately, even this definition does not completely neutralize need because the amount demanded at a zero price is likely to partly depend on a person's income. To the extent that medical care is a "normal" good, need, according to this definition, would vary positively with income, and it is by no means obvious, at least conceptually, that the poor would have unmet needs. Certainly, common sense suggests that they do.

The elusive nature of need has several implications for the analysis of our third dependent variable which is based on a question on unmet needs from the 1974 HIS. First, need is not fully objective from a medical vantage point, but rather reflects socioeconomic as well as medical factors. Certainly, this is true of an individual's patience with the speed according to which his needs are being met; the latter is also part of the notion of unmet needs. Second, there is no analytic framework that can immediately be applied to the notion of met and unmet needs. For this reason, regression analysis with this type of a dependent variable should be seen as a statistical description of responses to an oft-asked question rather than as an empirical evaluation of a theory of met and unmet needs.

Empirical Specification—The Explanatory Variables

Employment status and *income* represent explanatory variable categories of primary concern to this analysis. Employment status is represented by a set of binary variables. They are constructed on the basis of the household head's *usual* activity during the twelve months prior to the survey and his or her *current* activity, defined for the two-week period immediately prior to the survey. By "usual," the HIS means the status that best describes the person's activity during the past twelve months.

We have defined six employment status categories for our multivariate analysis of household head access. The first category consists of persons who usually worked during the preceding year and also worked during the two weeks prior to the survey. A second group is defined for persons who usually worked during the past year, and whose status during the last two weeks was not at work but with a job. This group consists of persons on layoffs as well as persons temporarily absent from work because of vacation, bad weather, labor disputes, and/or illness. On average, the second group may have had more "free" time at the time of the survey than the first group. Such persons may have had lower shadow wages and poor employment prospects, and may have experienced transitory income losses. However, most members of this group should still have the same job-related health insurance that they possessed prior to their work absences. A third group of household heads usually worked during the past year, but during the last two weeks, had no job. These persons comprise the group of short-term unemployed.

Fourth, there are household heads who usually did not work during the past year, but were employed during the past two weeks. These persons are the short-term employed. The short-term employed differ from the longer-term employed in several ways. The short-term employed may regard a large part of their current earnings as transitory rather than permanent. Such persons may not yet be fully eligible for health insurance offered by their employers. For example, exclusions pertaining to preexisting conditions may still apply. Finally, in answering questions regarding access during the past year, the short-term employed may respond more like unemployed than employed persons.

The long-term unemployed comprise the fifth employment status category. These heads usually had no job during the past year and were not employed during the past two weeks. Sixth, there are those household heads who were not usually employed during the last year and were out of the labor force during the two weeks' reference period. This category largely consists of retirees and female heads of household.

The six employment status groups are defined to be mutually exclusive. The choice of the excluded group for estimation purposes is necessary but arbitrary. We have excluded the first category—usually working, currently employed.[8]

Family size has a role quite similar to those of employment status and income. As family size increases, income and parental time per family member decreases. As per capita income decreases, the ability to purchase medical care and amenities associated with having a usual source of care concurrently decreases. However, as parental time availability decreases because parents are so busy consuming, they become more averse to waiting. It is impossible to speculate which of these forces will predominate on conceptual grounds alone.

Michael[9] and others have argued that education improves a person's performance as a consumer. In other words, given a fixed amount of income, more educated persons are able to secure greater amounts of goods and services because they are better negotiators in the marketplace, and they have a better ability to interpret many kinds of market information. If so, more schooling may be associated with better access, gauged in terms of a number of alternative measures. Since we thought that education would be highly collinear with other explanatory variables, especially employment status and income, we have estimated regressions with and without education. This variable is measured in terms of the number of years of schooling that the respondent completed.

As noted in chapter 2, several utilization studies have classified explanatory variables into predisposing, enabling, and need factors. Education falls into the predisposing category. Other variables in this category are sex, age, and race. Enabling variables include employment status, income, and family size. The enabling factors have received attention earlier in this chapter and we now address our concern to the predisposing factors.

Males and nonwhites are less likely to report a regular source of care than females and whites. Women, one can argue, are more apt to regularly visit a specialist, such as a gynecologist, and therefore are more likely than men to report a usual source of care. Moreover, with a usual source of care, women are more likely to experience continuity and encounter fewer problems obtaining care. We also expect that because of these differences, women, when compared to men, will be more satisfied with the care that they receive. The binary sex variable is one if the respondent is male.

Whereas children comprise the age group most likely to see a specialist (pediatrician) and therefore have one particular doctor as a usual source of care, this age group is excluded from our sample. For two of the three remaining age groups we have defined, young (25–44) and middle-aged (45–64), we do not have any reason to expect differential patterns regarding a usual source, problems obtaining care, and satisfaction; but we do not believe that older persons (65+) are more likely to have a particular doctor for two reasons. First, Medicare's coverage of physicians' services is relatively comprehensive. Second, because older persons are much more likely to have chronic conditions, the benefit from having a regular source is relatively great.

Due to discrimination and habit persistence (perhaps due to previous discrimination), one may anticipate that whites, compared to nonwhites, are more apt to report a regular source of care, fewer problems obtaining care, and more satisfaction with the care they receive. The binary race variable is one for white respondents.

In this chapter, need is represented by the presence of chronic conditions causing limitation of activity. The HIS defines four categories of activity limitation according to the extent to which activities are limited. These categories differentiate among persons who are unable to carry on a major activity, those not limited in a major activity but restricted in the amount or kind of major activity performed, those not limited in a major activity but otherwise limited, and those not limited in activities. Persons with very limiting chronic conditions are probably frequent users of physicians' services and are more likely to use regular sources. Whether they tend to be more satisfied with the level of care received and are less likely to encounter problems in obtaining care are issues to be settled empirically. Inasmuch as this variable implies only the presence of chronic or long-term conditions, we expect that the employment status variable might also partially reflect need by representing short-term or stress-induced, acute limitations of activities. The four activity limitation categories are defined to be mutually exclusive. One of these, household heads without an activity limitation, is the omitted group.

Finally, variables are included in the access regressions to represent community size and regional influences. Two separate studies, Sloan and Berry, et al., found that the time that patients spend obtaining ambulatory care (travel time plus waiting time) is higher in the most heavily populated cities.[10] Although these studies support the previously stated expectation of a negative relationship between the physician-population ratio and patient time, they find that the ratio per se explains relatively little of the total intercommunity variation in patient time. The evidence from these studies implies that there are substantial geographical disparities in the patient's time input; moreover, with the exception of the Farm-South, rural farm communities do not require as much aggregated travel and waiting time as several major cities. Our expectation is to discern similar trends in access. Consequently, we anticipate a positive association between the proportion of our sample which lives in central cities and the propensity to report that they encounter many problems—and little satisfaction—with their access to medical care. Our community size variables are: SMSA Central City;[11] SMSA NonCentral City; NonSMSA; NonFarm; and Farm. Household heads living on farms are the omitted group.

Regional effects are represented by binary variables for the Census Areas—Northeast, North Central, South, and West, the omitted category. Area price and insurance variables are two enabling variables that have been considered for use in this analysis, but were not included in this chapter's empirical work. We decided not to attempt to merge price information with the HIS data base because, with the exception of the largest SMSAs, communities are not identified. A limited amount of insurance information is available from the 1974 HIS, but merging this information with the access responses would have been very costly. Since insurance coverage is not explicitly considered, we expect the partial effect of insurance to be partly reflected in the estimated parameters for employment status, family income, and the regional variables. It is known, for example, that fewer persons have private health insurance coverage in the West, holding a large number of factors constant.[12] The following two chapters explicitly consider both area price and insurance variables.

Table 4-2 contains a list of explanatory variables with sample means, standard deviations, and concise definitions. This table describes our sample;

Table 4-2
Access of Household Heads: Means, Standard Deviations, and Definitions

Variable	Mean	Standard Deviation	Definition
Sex	0.791	0.406	Respondent is male (= 1).
Young	0.449	0.497	Respondent is 25–44 years old (= 1).
Middle-aged	0.348	0.477	Respondent is 45–64 years old (= 1).
Race	0.896	0.306	Respondent is white (= 1).
Family income	12.554	7.912	Respondent's family income from all sources (in thousands of dollars).
Education	11.4	3.7	Years of schooling completed by respondent.
Northeast	0.238	0.426	Respondent lives in either Maine, New Hampshire, Vermont, Massachusetts, Rhode Island, Connecticut, New York, New Jersey, Pennsylvania (= 1).
North central	0.267	0.443	Respondent lives in Michigan, Ohio, Indiana, Illinois, Wisconsin, Minnesota, Iowa, Missouri, North Dakota, South Dakota, Nebraska, or Kansas (= 1).
South	0.306	0.461	Respondent lives in Delaware, Maryland, District of Columbia, Virginia, West Virginia, North Carolina, South Carolina, Georgia, Florida, Kentucky, Texas, Tennessee, Alabama, Mississippi, Arkansas, Louisiana, or Oklahoma (= 1).
SMSA, Central city	0.305	0.460	Respondent lives within the Central City of a Standard Metropolitan Area (SMSA) (= 1).
SMSA, Noncentral city	0.385	0.487	Respondent lives within a SMSA, outside of the central city (= 1).
NonSMSA, nonfarm	0.275	0.447	Respondent lives outside of a SMSA, but not on a farm (= 1).
Usually working, with job, but not at work now	0.014	0.177	Respondent is usually (most of the time within the last 12 months) working, had job but not at work during the last 2 weeks (= 1).
Working, usually working, but no job now	0.012	0.110	Respondent is usually working but had no job in last 2 weeks (= 1).
Usually not working, but now at work	0.022	0.145	Respondent is usually not working, but at work in last 2 weeks (= 1).

Usually not working, and now not at work	0.011	0.102	Respondent is usually not working and unemployed in last 2 weeks (= 1).
Not in labor force	0.198	0.399	Respondent has been neither employed nor unemployed either in last year or last 2 weeks (= 1)
Family size	2.74	2.01	Number of family members.
Cannot perform activity	0.054	0.226	Respondent is unable to carry on major activity, such as work (= 1).
Limited usual activity	0.100	0.300	Respondent is limited in the amount or kind of major activity performed (= 1).
Limited outside activity	0.051	0.221	Respondent is not limited in major activity but is otherwise limited (= 1).

as previously mentioned, our sample is limited to heads of households; it is comprised of a substantial proportion (nearly 20 percent) of females. Nearly one fifth of our sample is over age 65;[13] approximately 10 percent is nonwhite, and nearly one-third of our sample resides in the South. Very few household heads included in our analysis (3.5 percent) live on a farm.

Considering employment status, nearly 20 percent of our sample is not in the labor force. The unemployment rate of heads in our sample (calculated by summing the proportions of each category of unemployed persons including the "layoff" category) is 3.7 percent. This rate is substantially lower than the 1974 national unemployment rate, reflecting the tendency for the "secondary" workers and youths (persons below age 25) to have higher than average unemployment rates. The latter types of persons are excluded from our sample.

Estimation

Our dependent variables are binary and can therefore only assume two different values, zero and one. Specifically, we attempt to explain the likelihood for people to have a regular source of care, to experience problems in obtaining care, and to receive as much care as needed. In technical terms, these are linear probability models. The estimated coefficients express the probability that a "one" will be observed, given the levels of the explanatory variables.

When ordinary least squares (OLS) are used in this context, one obtains unbiased, but inefficient (less precise), parameter estimates. Furthermore, predicted probabilities may fall outside the zero-one interval. Several techniques have been developed to deal with one or both of these statistical problems, for example, probit and logit analysis, and weighted OLS.[14] Weighted regressions deal with inefficiency, and we have used the weights provided by HIS for this purpose. It is possible that a few predictions from our regressions would fall outside the zero-one interval, but prediction per se is not an important objective of this chapter. Since we desire to gauge the impacts of employment status on access, we need to use all 8,656 valid observations on household heads.[15] Maximum likelihood techniques, including probit and logit analysis, are very expensive when applied to samples of this size.

Empirical Results

Table 4-3 presents our regressions. Although the overall explanatory power of our equations, as measured by $R^2 s$, is very low, our results are useful for assessing the statistical significance of particular variables, as well as the signs and magnitudes of the effects of the explanatory variables. Low $R^2 s$ are common in regressions based on micro units (for instance, individuals), but the $R^2 s$ in table

Table 4–3
Access of Household Heads: Regression Results

Variable	Usual Source		Any Problem Obtaining Care		Receiving as Much Care as Needed
Sex	−0.111 (0.014)*	−0.110 (0.014)*	−0.055 (0.009)*	−0.054 (0.009)*	0.020 (0.009)*
Young	−0.093 (0.066)	−0.096 (0.066)	0.116 (0.050)†	0.108 (0.050)†	−0.071 (0.043)‡
Middle-aged	0.007 (0.066)	0.0050 (0.066)	0.067 (0.050)	0.064 (0.050)	−0.058 (0.043)
Race	0.022 (0.014)	0.020 (0.016)	0.022 (0.011)†	0.018 (0.011)‡	0.049 (0.009)*
Family income	0.0041 (0.0006)*	0.0038 (0.0007)*	−0.0010 (0.0005)‡	−0.0015 (0.0006)*	0.0022 (0.0004)*
Education	− (−)	0.0016 (0.0014)	− (−)	0.0029 (0.0011)*	− (−)
Northeast	0.020 (0.014)	0.021 (0.014)	−0.038 (0.009)*	−0.037 (0.010)*	0.022 (0.009)*
North Central	0.070 (0.014)*	0.070 (0.014)*	−0.021 (0.009)†	−0.020 (0.010)†	0.030 (0.009)*
South	0.031 (0.014)†	0.033 (0.014)†	−0.020 (0.009)†	−0.018 (0.009)‡	0.010 (0.009)
SMSA, Central City	−0.042 (0.025)‡	−0.044 (0.025)‡	0.038 (0.018)†	0.035 (0.018)‡	−0.002 (0.016)
SMSA, noncentral city	0.016 (0.025)	−0.018 (0.025)	0.042 (0.018)†	0.038 (0.018)†	0.003 (0.016)
NonSMSA, nonfarm	−0.011 (0.025)	−0.011 (0.025)	0.038 (0.018)†	0.036 (0.018)‡	0.023 (0.016)
Usually working, with job, but not at work now	0.084 (0.036)†	0.084 (0.036)†	0.034 (0.027)	0.034 (0.027)	0.000 (0.025)
Usually working, but no job now	−0.156 (0.039)*	−0.156 (0.039)*	0.103 (0.030)*	0.104 (0.030)*	−0.060 (0.025)†
Usually not working, but now at work	0.022 (0.030)	0.020 (0.030)	0.070 (0.023)*	0.070 (0.023)*	−0.025 (0.020)
Usually not working and now not at work	−0.095 (0.043)†	−0.097 (0.043)†	0.111 (0.032)*	0.107 (0.032)*	−0.076 (0.027)*
Not in labor force	0.049 (0.066)	0.049 (0.066)	0.023 (0.050)	0.023 (0.050)	−0.017 (0.043)
Family size	0.012 (0.002)*	0.013 (0.002)*	−0.002 (0.002)	−0.001 (0.002)	−0.004 (0.002)‡
Cannot perform activity	0.124 (0.023)*	0.125 (0.023)*	0.124 (0.018)*	0.127 (0.018)*	−0.068 (0.014)*
Limited usual activity	0.065 (0.016)*	0.066 (0.016)*	0.073 (0.011)*	0.074 (0.011)*	−0.078 (0.009)*

Table 4–3 continued

Variable	Usual Source		Any Problem Obtaining Care		Receiving as Much Care as Needed
Limited outside activity	0.066 (0.020)*	0.067 (0.020)*	0.076 (0.016)*	0.076 (0.016)*	−0.053 (0.014)*
Constant	0.0773 (−)	0.761 (−)	0.030 (−)	0.009 (−)	0.896 (−)
	$R^2 = 0.05$	$R^2 = 0.05$	$R^2 = 0.03$	$R^2 = 0.03$	$R^2 = 0.03$
	$F(20,8636)$ = 116.6	$F(21,8635)$ = 111.4*	$F(21,8635)$ = 67.9*	$F(21,8636)$ = 66.5*	$F(20,8635)$ = 66.0*

*Significant at the 1 percent level; †significant at the 5 percent level; ‡significant at the 10 percent level.

4-3 are low by even these standards. Nevertheless, the majority of parameter estimates in the table are statistically significant at the 10 percent level (two-tail test) or better. We shall discuss regressions on each of the three dependent variables separately.

Family income has the anticipated positive effect on the likelihood of having a usual source of care, and the coefficient is statistically significant. The parameter estimates imply that a $10,000 decrease in family income would lower the probability of possessing a usual source by about 0.04. Corresponding elasticities (evaluated at the sample means) are in the −0.06 to −0.07 range.

The two "no job" categories have anticipated negative coefficients and they are statistically significant, but it is difficult to explain why the short-term unemployed are less likely to have regular sources than the long-term unemployed. As discussed below, the long-term unemployed fare slightly worse in terms of the other two access measures. If the $10,000 income loss is combined with the long-term unemployment, a likely combination if unemployment persists, the parameter estimates imply that the probability of having a usual source falls by about 0.14.

Judged in terms of statistical significance, the short-term employed and non-labor force participants are about as likely to have a regular source as are employed heads. We are not able to explain why the "with job, but not now at work" group, which includes heads on layoff, has a greater likelihood of possessing a usual source than employed persons in general. The family size coefficient is positive and significant in the usual source regressions. As noted above, the direction of effect could not be predicted on conceptual grounds alone.

Education, when included, has a positive impact, but the associated elasticity is low (0.02). Including this variable has virtually no effect on the other parameter estimates. Of the remaining predisposing variables, only the sex coefficients are statistically significant. The results imply that males are 0.11 less likely to have a usual source. Unlike the regressions for the other two dependent variables, the difference between whites and nonwhites is small and statistically insignificant.

The result that household heads with activity limitations are more likely to have usual sources of care is reassuring from the standpoint of policy. The result that residents of central cities of SMSAs are less likely to have usual sources supports the aforementioned finding that travel and office waiting time are also higher in these communities. Persons in the West are least likely to have a regular source; individuals located in the North Central Census Area are the most likely to have one, holding other factors constant.

The results for the second dependent variable are broadly consistent with those for the first, but there are a few notable exceptions. In interpreting the findings, one must recall that, as defined, the first and third dependent variables represent "goods" while having a problem obtaining care is a "bad." A negative coefficient implies better access when the dependent variable refers to a bad.

The income and employment status coefficients imply that the poor and the long-term unemployed have above-average chances of encountering a problem. Although the coefficients on the income variables are lower in absolute value than in the usual source regressions, the associated elasticities are more than twice as great (ranging from 0.11 to 0.18). The contrast in the elasticities reflect the fact that elasticities are evaluated at different means (of the dependent variable). Combining a loss of $10,000 with long-term unemployment, the probability of encountering a problem rises by 0.12. Short-term unemployment also raises the likelihood of an access problem, but the increase is slightly less than for the long-term unemployed.

The positive and significant coefficient on the education variable is surprising. Perhaps more highly educated persons have greater expectations and thus tend to report problems that others would not mention. However, while the argument seems plausible for the second dependent variable, education demonstrates absolutely no impact on the unmet needs variable. If expectations are indeed higher, the more educated should also have been more likely to complain about unmet needs. Education was highly insignificant in the needs regression, which is not reported.

Although household heads with health limitations are more likely to have usual sources, they also tend to encounter more problems obtaining care. Furthermore, in contrast to the usual source regressions, whites are more likely to report problems, but racial differences are quite small. As above, residents of farms have better access, but using the problems dependent variable, access of household heads living in central cities is no worse than it is for household heads in other nonfarm locations.

The unmet need regression also implies that low income and unemployed heads have worse access. The associated income elasticity, however, is quite low (0.03). The long-term unemployed are slightly more likely to report unmet needs than the short-term unemployed; the coefficients are, respectively, −0.076 and −0.060. As with the usual source, but unlike the problems dependent variable, whites have fewer unmet needs than non-whites.

Many of the results from our regressions with "any problem obtaining care" and "receiving as much care as needed" are consistent with the results of a cross-tabular analysis based on 1975 Medical Access Study data.[16] For example, conclusions with regard to income and race are reinforced. But the cross-tabular analysis implies that persons in the South are least satisfied with care received, and more educated persons tend to be satisfied. We know that education and family income are highly correlated; possibly, education picked up the effect of income in the cross-tabular study. As we have said, we find a small income effect on satisfaction with care received. Cross-tabular studies often look for differences but give insufficient emphasis to the size of these differences.

Summary, Conclusions, and Implications

This chapter presents the results of empirical work on selected qualitative aspects of medical care utilization. From our results, we conclude that the type of care that individuals receive is partially related to prevailing economic conditions. In contrast to chapter 3, where we focused on utilization, in this chapter we stressed the process and satisfaction dimension of access with data from the 1974 Health Interview Survey (HIS). Although the 1974 HIS is a single cross-section, we have used it to generate some time-related inferences. First, we compared responses to access questions obtained from respondents during the first quarter of 1974 with those obtained in the fourth quarter of that year. Since the economy deteriorated rapidly during 1974, we would have been not at all surprised to observe a deterioration in at least some dimensions of access; however, no meaningful changes were evident. Second, the regression analysis has allowed us to gauge differential effects of short- versus long-term unemployment on access. We find the long-term unemployed to be worse off in terms of both experiencing problems obtaining care and receiving as much care as needed.

We have presented cross-tabulations on several process and satisfaction measures of access by family income and current (as of the 1974 interview) employment status. By and large, these tabulations show unemployed and low income persons to have poorer access. Such persons are more likely to have no usual source of care, to encounter various problems obtaining care, and to have unmet health needs. Cross-tabulations are easy to interpret, at least superficially, but they also have important limitations. In our context, the percentage differences among the cells in our tables are small; the tables contrast current employment with current unemployment with no reference to the duration of either. Of course, with two-way tables, there is always a lingering suspicion that some "other" factor (or factors) is really responsible for the observed differences.

Given the limitations of the cross-tabulations, we have performed regression analysis on three access variables: whether or not the respondent has a usual source of care; whether or not he has encountered problems obtaining care; and whether or not he has unmet medical needs.

The regressions again imply that the poor and the unemployed are worse off. Unemployment and income loss taken together account for a meaningful loss in access, about 10 percentage points, assuming a $5,000 drop in annual income. We have included educational attainment as an explanatory variable in some of our regressions. Education never disturbs the relationship between income-employment status on the one hand and access to physicians' services on the other.

The regressions show differences in access on the basis of race, but non-whites are not always worse off. Persons with activity limitations are more likely to have a usual source of care; but they are also more likely to encounter problems obtaining care and to have unmet health needs. Certainly, one cannot gauge access in toto from evidence on one access measure.

Although our results imply that adverse effects on access should be included in any itemization of the costs of unemployment, our results also suggest that the elimination of these unemployment-induced adverse effects on access would not appreciably improve the nation's access to medical care. We find that although most of the included variables have the anticipated impact on access, the set of variables included in our analysis explains little of the total interpersonal variation in access, as measured by R^2s. Thus, if public policies greatly reduced unemployment, there is no reason to expect that the access differentials would be very different from those observed during a recession year in the mid-1970s. A full-employment strategy is simply not enough.

Notes

1. The public use of tapes offer much more information on general access-related issues than we present here. Some more general findings are found in Joel C. Kleinman and Ronald W. Wilson, "Are Medically Under-Served Areas' Medically Underserved?" *Health Services Research* 12 (Summer 1977):147–162, and will be reported by the NCHS in official publications.

2. Lu Ann Aday and Ronald Andersen, *Access to Medical Care,* Ann Arbor, Michigan: Health Administration Press, 1975.

3. Harold S. Luft, John C. Hershey, and Joan Morrell, "Factors Affecting the Use of Physician Services in a Rural Community," *American Journal of Public Health* 66 (September 1976):865–871. 1974; David Salkever, "Economic Class and Differential Access to Care: Comparison Among Health Care Systems," *International Journal of Health Services* 5 (Summer 1975):373–95.

4. The percents under "place of usual care" add to 80.4 in the first column of table 4-3.

5. Department of Health, Education and Welfare, National Center for Health Statistics, *Interviewer's Manual, 1974 Health Interview Survey,* (processed), p. 28.

6. To some extent, this tendency of the unemployed to rely on insurance reflects the lack of available payors, such as Workmen's Compensation.

7. For a discussion of the merit want concept, see Richard A. Musgrave, *The Theory of Public Finance,* New York: McGraw-Hill, 1959.

8. Two issues related to employment status deserve attention. First, all three dependent variables, though sometimes reflective of objective circumstances, are based on respondent perceptions. There may be important lags in perceptions. For instance, suppose a person has been unemployed for two months and is asked about his usual source of care. Once such a person actually decides to use health services, he may change providers. But since he has not sought medical advice or treatment in the past two months, his response may reflect circumstances before he lost his job. This notion of lags may even be more pertinent in the case of the other two dependent variables. To the extent that perceptions lag, we shall overstate the short-term effects of job loss. Dependent variables in other chapters refer to actual occurrences and hence are not subject to this particular problem. Second, family income is also included as an explanatory variable, and, therefore, the income and employment status variables jointly share the influence of economic conditions. Income information for the twelve months preceding the survey was requested. In many cases, 1973 income information may have been given instead. If so, the employment status variables would often provide better measures of short-term income changes.

9. Robert T. Michael, "Education in Nonmarket Production," *Journal of Political Economy* 81 (March–April 1973):306-327.

10. See Frank Sloan, "Access to Medical Care and the Local Supply of Physicians," *Medical Care* 18 (April 1977):338-346 and Charles Berry et al., Report on the Physician Capacity Utilization Survey, Final Report on Rand Subcontract No. 75-39, *Mathematica Policy Research,* January 30, 1976.

11. A central city includes the largest city in the SMSA and, in some cases, additional comparatively large cities within the SMSA. This concept of central city is different from the usual connotation of central city which refers to the community's inner area. The remainder of the SMSA, likely to be largely suburban, is classified as SMSA Noncentral City.

12. Frank Sloan and Bruce Steinwald, *Hospital Costs and Input Choices: Effects of Insurance, Regulation, and Other Factors,* unpublished.

13. This is determined by adding the fractions young and middle-aged and subtracting the resulting sum from one.

14. See Jan Kmenta, *Elements of Econometrics,* New York: Collier-MacMillan, 1971.

15. The access supplement to the 1974 HIS was only administered to a sub-sample of HIS respondents.

16. The Robert Wood Johnson Foundation, *Special Report on Access—America's Health Care System: A Comprehensive Portrait,* Princeton, New Jersey, 1978.

5 Demand for Ambulatory Care in Alternative Practice Settings

Students of qualitative aspects of the delivery of physicians' services have emphasized differences by practice setting and physician specialty in continuity of patient care, in physicians' ability to render care appropriate to particular nonmedical conditions, in patient waiting time at the site of care, and in emergency or quasi-emergency situations, immediate patient access to medical care. Many informed observers contend that hospital-based providers are less likely to offer continuity of patient care and management of comprehensive family care than are private (or office-based) physicians.[1] This factor is important since information costs involved in obtaining pertinent background data, both medical and nonmedical, at each visit are substantial. Consequently, some questions that may ultimately prove to be relevant to the outcome of treatment may never be asked.

As noted in chapter 3, the share of total visits to physicians that are visits to hospital outpatient departments (OPD) and emergency rooms (ER) has increased during the 1970s. During the last year for which data are available, 1975, the OPD-ER share of total visits was at its peak. The growth in the OPD-ER share was higher than usual during 1974–1975, the inflation-recession years. Finally, the dependence of low-income persons on the OPD and ER for physicians' services, as measured by the OPD-ER share, is far greater than the average. It has been estimated that one-third to two-thirds of emergency room care is of a nonemergency nature.[2]

The tendency for patients to wait longer in waiting rooms of hospital-based providers is well documented.[3] Hence, persons who have high shadow wages should be more likely, holding other factors constant, to eschew care from hospital sources. There is also evidence from previous research that persons who seek appointments at hospital outpatient departments experience greater delays in obtaining care than patients of office-based physicians.[4]

Another oft-cited criticism of the U.S. medical care system is that too many kinds of health conditions are treated by specialists rather than generalist physicians. As a result, too many specialized procedures, including surgery, are performed.[5] Specialists, however, are thought to be more productive and effective in treating many conditions that occur frequently. To the extent that the demand for specialists is more responsive to patient income than is the demand for physicians in general, adverse economic conditions that lead to income losses, actual and anticipated, and loss of insurance coverage may have the salutary effect of reducing the use of specialists in cases when general physicians could render as good or perhaps even better care.

In this chapter we investigate and analyze patterns of patient choice of provider setting. Alternatives considered are visits by persons over age 25 to either: (1) a general practitioner in a private office; (2) a specialist in a private office; (3) a hospital outpatient department; or (4) an emergency room. Determinants of patients' choices are assessed using discriminant analysis.

General-family practitioners, general internists, and general pediatricians, the groups most often classified as general or primary care physicians, ideally would be responsible for overall patient management, except perhaps when the patient has an unusual medical condition. Thus, ideally, we would have distinguished between physicians who provide primary care and physicians who do not, rather than between general practitioners and specialists. Unfortunately, our data base does not permit one to determine whether an internist is "general"; and, as a result, all internists are considered to be specialists. Since the analysis in this and the following chapter is confined to adults, visits to pediatricians do not apply.

In chapter 6 we examine sources of variation in some of the process variables thought to vary systematically with the provider setting—patient waiting time, length-of-visit, and appointment delays. The analysis in this chapter and that in chapter 6 are based on the Medical Access Study, a national survey of the U.S. population conducted during the latter part of 1975 by the University of Chicago. The analyses in chapters 5 and 6 use a common set of explanatory variables.[6]

There are several principal policy issues to be investigated in these two chapters.

1. As emphasized in chapter 1, there is reason to expect that the opportunity wage is lower for unemployed persons, holding other factors constant. As the opportunity wage and income fall, it is reasonable to expect patients to select sources of care which require a lower money price even if a greater time input is demanded. Therefore, we hypothesize that waiting time at the site of care is higher for jobless persons, and sources of care associated with longer waiting time, for example, hospital outpatient departments and emergency rooms are used more frequently. Patient waiting may yield cost savings in the production of ambulatory care; the substitution of less expensive patient time for more expensive provider time may be economically (allocatively) efficient, given that people are unemployed. Such substitutions, however, may be viewed by policy makers as undesirable on equity grounds.

2. As noted in chapter 1, it appears that retired persons and public assistance recipients on average maintained their real incomes during 1974–1975. However, families experiencing job loss undoubtedly lost real income. To the extent that the qualitative dimensions of access considered in chapters 4, 5, and 6 are "normal goods" (are demanded in greater amounts as real income rises),

they should be in less demand during cyclical downturns in the economy. For this reason, we evaluate the strength of the ("pure") income effects, both permanent and transitory, on each of the dependent variables. If the levels of these access measures do depend on real income, one could legitimately count improved access to ambulatory care as one of the benefits from increasing the levels of unemployment and/or public assistance payments. We already have cited evidence in chapter 3 of a strong impact of income on the use of physicians' services, and a significant, albeit small, impact of income of the process and satisfaction measures, assessed in chapter 4.

3. Lee estimated that the loss of private group health insurance coincident with the loss of employment is substantial.[7] Although the fact that health insurance subsidizes utilization is now widely understood, insurance also frequently subsidizes the qualitative features of a visit. This is seen most directly in the case of major medical insurance, the predominant form of private insurance for (nonsurgical) office visits to physicians. Major medical insurance usually pays 75 to 80 percent of a "reasonable" fee. To the extent that third-party payors consider high fees associated with the purchase of high quality-amenity visits to be reasonable, reimbursements are higher than when lower quality-amenity levels are selected.[8] Unemployed persons who lose their private insurance are no longer eligible for this subsidy, and therefore may turn to less expensive sources of care.

Proposals for extending health insurance protection to the unemployed were proposed in Congress during 1975.[9] Unemployment rates have fallen somewhat since then and there is currently no strong interest in such legislation. However, if such legislation were to be reconsidered, estimates of the impact of third-party coverage on various access dimensions would provide a needed element for evaluating its payoffs. In chapter 3, our insurance measure, the percentage of total expenditures on physicians' services reimbursed by private and public third parties, demonstrated no effect on utilization. In part, the insignificant effect of the insurance variable may be attributed to the small amount of variation in coverage in our time series and to multicollinearity. There is merit in further assessing the impact of insurance with cross-sectional data in this and the following chapter.

4. The adverse economic conditions of 1974–1975 resulted in increased citizen dependence on Medicaid.[10] A recent study of physician participation in Medicaid programs showed that participation of office-based physicians in Medicaid is highly dependent on Medicaid reimbursement levels, reimbursement levels of private third-party payors, and bureaucratic problems the physician often faces in dealing with Medicaid.[11] If physicians who offer high levels of various amenities and charge high fees for these services refuse to participate in Medicaid, which tends to pay less than other third-party payors,[12] Medicaid patients will be forced to obtain "second class" care from physicians who do not offer these amenities. In this chapter, we attempt to ascertain whether this is so. In the next chapter, we shall determine whether Medicaid recipients have to wait

longer, experience longer appointment delays and have shorter visits than other persons.

5. The relatively high rates of unemployment among blacks and Spanish-surnamed individuals are well documented. Recessions tend to have a disproportionate impact on ethnic minorities. Such persons are among the first to be terminated during recessions. Inequalities in job markets are only one kind of inequity these minorities face. A recent study by Sloan reported that blacks have a higher propensity to use hospital-based physicians, holding other factors constant.[13] Sloan and Lorant[14] found that blacks, holding such factors of income constant, tend to wait longer than whites once they have arrived at the site of care, but no differences were found in Sloan and Lorant's regression analysis of variations in length of visit.[15] In chapter 4, small race effects were reported, but whites did not always have an advantage. Since our regressions, like previous studies, contain ability-to-pay variables, any differentials in access attributable to race and ethnicity must reflect a lack of physicians in areas in which minorities work and live, outright discrimination, and/or preference differences. The last of these explanations is the least plausible by far, but it cannot be ruled out on the basis of the evidence presented.

6. Physician manpower policies are largely justified in terms of improved access to ambulatory care. But until recently there has been surprisingly little empirical research on the nexus between physician availability and access. Our failure to find significant impacts of physician availability on utilization in the time series analysis outlined in chapter 3 should not discourage further inquiry into the effects of physician availability on access.

The plan of this chapter is as follows. In the next section we will discuss conceptual considerations pertinent to the study of patient choice of provider type. We then briefly describe the data base used in this and the following chapter. Next, we set out the empirical specification of our provider choice model and report our empirical results. In the final section we summarize our findings.

Conceptual Framework

In the pioneering work of Grossman, the household possesses a utility function with health and a composite variable representing other commodities as arguments.[16] Health in turn is produced by the household using purchased units of medical care, time, including exercise, good health habits (for instance, no smoking or excessive alcohol consumption), and other variables as inputs. The demand for medical care is derived from a more basic demand for health. Using this approach, both the patient's health status and various inputs, including his use of different types of health services, are endogenous to the model.

Although we will retain the spirit of this model in terms of many of the included exogenous variables, an assessment of practice setting does require certain departures. First, the Grossman model does not consider stochastic changes in health status, which must be counted as a potentially important determinant of practice setting choice.[17] An unexpected deviation from one's "normal" or previous health state is one reason for using an emergency room. Certain chronic conditions are probably best treated by specialists. It would be virtually impossible, and given the principal objectives of this study undesirable, to develop an operational model to explain a person's health state at a single point in time. Thus, we treat the health state at the time of visit as exogenous. Second, Grossman assumed that the patient time input in the consumption of a unit of medical care is fixed. As we have said, there is evidence that patients wait longer in clinics and emergency rooms than in private physicians' offices. In our work, patient time itself is a decision variable. Third, Grossman's model does not explicitly consider amenities or disamenities associated with the consumption of medical services that do not directly contribute to improvements in health. A person's choice of provider type, however, may be very much influenced by the levels and kinds of amenities offered in various settings, even though these amenities do not directly contribute to better health.

It must be emphasized that Grossman's simplifying assumptions were made for analytic convenience, and they allowed him to derive results using formal methods. As each assumption is relaxed, the model becomes much more complex and difficult to work with on a formal basis. More generalized versions become impossible to solve analytically. Therefore, we proceed on an intuitive rather than on a formal basis.

We assume, for example, that persons with comparatively high shadow wages choose providers who do not require them to wait long; furthermore, we assume that various amenities associated with the receipt of care are normal goods. Therefore, as nonearned as well as earned income rises, patients are more likely, *ceteris paribus,* to select physicians who offer various kinds of amenities. To the extent, for instance, that people have a distaste for waiting per se, short waits too may be seen as a normal good.

Our modification of previous work is crucial for interpreting both this and the following chapter and, for this reason, merits further discussion. Time is likely to be important to patients for two reasons. First, time devoted to ambulatory care cannot be allocated to other uses. Second, many patients do not find time spent in or traveling to the physician's office especially enjoyable. The economic theory of the household, developed by Becker[18] and others, readily takes the first of these factors into account. It predicts that persons with high shadow wages will demand, holding other factors constant, goods and services requiring comparatively low consumer time inputs. Given several varieties of a particular good or service the consumer will select the one requiring the least consumer time. For example, faced with the option of flying or sailing to Europe, the person with the higher shadow wage is more likely, holding other factors constant, to fly. Likewise, he is more likely to choose a physician who does not make his patients wait, even if he has to pay more out of pocket.

Although economists recognize the importance of the latter factor, it has not generally been incorporated in their research, which typically has stressed the role of time price. If one measured the shadow wages of persons flying and sailing to Europe, it is certainly possible that transoceanic ship passengers might well have higher shadow wages on the average. Consider the consumption benefits associated with sailing. If time were the only consideration, jet travel would certainly be preferred, but it is clearly not the only consideration. Various amenities on ships yield benefits in their own right. If waiting for the doctor is distasteful, the relatively affluent would try to reduce their time input as a means of reducing their discomfort, much as they purchase air conditioning to free them from the heat or buy a luxurious automobile for its smooth and quiet ride. If patients find waiting distasteful, the shadow wage understates the cost of waiting. How much it is understated is unfortunately an empirical question that this or any study has yet to answer.

Waiting time at the site of care, appointment delays, and length of visit all involve patient time, but this is most obvious in the case of waiting time. A patient denied immediate access to a physician must lose time from work, recreation, or some other leisure activity. However, this is not usually an important factor. Longer waits require more patient time as well as more provider time. Still, the potential marginal benefit from increased contact usually outweighs the marginal patient time cost. More immediate access and lengthier visits are likely to be seen as desirable features in their own right, quite apart from the time element involved. Continuity of care has essentially nothing to do with patient time, but it is plausible to assume that it too is a normal good.

The access regressions specified and estimated below contain measures of the individual's shadow wage and their measured income. The shadow wage, of course, is equivalent to the opportunity cost of time. As the value of unit of time increases, the individual is expected to reduce the amount of his or her time input in the consumption of physicians' services. At the same time, high-wage persons and those with a lot of unearned income tend to be wealthier and therefore to demand various amenities in greater amounts. For this reason, one would expect that waiting time should fall and length of visit should rise with increases in income.

Our regressions, based on samples of married persons, contain the wage of the household head and that of the spouse. According to the economic theory of the household, family members capable of earning a high-market wage will specialize in market work while those with lower market wage are more prone to specialize in household work. High-wage persons are also more likely to consume goods and services requiring less of their time. Accordingly, if anyone in the household is to receive priority in obtaining low patient wait services from physicians, it will be the family member with the highest earning potential in the marketplace. This theory implies the waiting times of members of the same household would not be the same unless their wages were the same.

It is essential to recognize that empirical research on the economic theory of the household is still in its infancy. Although there is a substantial body of evidence that labor force decisions are made on the basis of comparative earning power, there is currently very little empirical support for or against the view that intrafamily consumption patterns depend on relative time prices of family members.

The role of insurance is more straightforward. Health insurance, especially major medical insurance, subsidizes both the quantity and quality of physicians' services. Medicaid, however, constitutes an important exception. Fee schedules tend to be low and supplementation by patient out-of-pocket payments is not allowed. For these reasons, some physicians may tend to "skimp" in the delivery of care to these patients.

Data

The Medical Access Study (MAS) was conducted by the National Opinion Research Center (NORC) of the University of Chicago for the University's Center for Health Administration Studies (CHAS) during the latter part of 1975. The MAS is an outgrowth of four previous national household surveys of health care utilization and expenditures, the last of which was conducted in 1971.[19]

The primary purpose of the MAS was to provide reliable estimates on several dimensions of access to medical care. The sponsor of the survey was the Robert Wood Johnson Foundation of Princeton, New Jersey. The National Center for Health Services Research provided additional funding to CHAS for additional data analysis.

The MAS consists of face-to-face interviews with 5,432 households, and 7,787 persons within these households. The survey is an area probability sample with all of NORC's 104 Primary Sampling Units (*PSUs*) plus two oversamples, a black oversample in the South and a Spanish heritage oversample in the Southwest. We have not attempted to reweigh the sample for purposes of analysis for two reasons. First, as discussed below and more fully in the appendix, we used two-limit probit analysis (TLP) in attempts to derive shadow wage measures and our TLP program does not contain a weighted regression routine. Second, since our access regressions are estimated separately for several population groups, after applying various screens, only Spanish-surnamed individuals are slightly overrepresented in some access regressions.[20]

A number of area variables from the U.S. Bureau of Health Manpower have been merged with the MAS by *PSU,* including the physician-population ratios used in our regressions. Also, diagnoses have been classified according to the degree of acuteness and severity by a panel of physicians, a psychologist, and a medical intern. Our use of the MAS diagnosis classification is described more fully below.

Empirical Specification

The nature of the variables included in the analysis of provider choice and, when possible, their anticipated effect on patient choice of provider are discussed in this section. Further detail on the specification of the income-employment variables is presented in the appendix.

Samples

We performed discriminant analysis on four samples of individuals: (1) female heads of households aged 25 to 64; (2) married men aged 25 to 64; (3) married women aged 25 to 64; and (4) retired persons over age 65 living in families with a husband and wife present. There are two reasons for stratifying. First, equation specification depends on family structure. Retiree regressions do not contain explanatory variables representing the opportunity cost of time. Medicare only pertains to persons over age 65. Variables representing the spouse's wage are irrelevant for female heads of household. Second, there is reason to expect differences in responses to particular explanatory variables, such as those describing the medical reasons for the visit.

Dependent Variable

The provider choice analysis based on samples of married persons considers the four alternatives specified above. Our female head and retiree samples are substantially smaller, and for this reason, we combine hospital outpatient and emergency room visits in these cases.

Information on the dependent variables pertains to the respondent's most recent visit to a physician. Alternatively, we could have considered information related to the patient's usual source of care. We selected visit-specific data because a significant fraction of the poor do not have a usual source. Also, we learned in the process of developing our own instrument to measure patient access that many persons have more than one usual source. Thus, for example, one person might consider both an internist and a gynecologist to be usual sources. Moreover, it is reasonable to expect that provider choice will be sensitive to the medical reason for a particular visit. Over time, a patient may see a physician, or physicians, for different reasons, and there is no way to accommodate such variation with information pertinent to the individual's usual source.

Money Price

Although the MAS includes insurance information, respondents were not queried about fees charged.[21] Nor is there any reliable information from any other source for 1975, or any recent year, on fees charged by alternative providers by geographic area. Fortunately, there is no particular reason to expect area prices to be systematically related on the whole to the other independent variables which, with the one exception of the area physician-population ratios, are measured at the level of the individual respondent. Therefore, there is little basis for anticipating omitted variables bias. But it is possible, and in fact likely, that fees of hospital-based physicians in particular reflect the respondent's ability to pay.[22] If so, the fee facing the individual would be lower for poorly insured and low-income persons. One can show that this second factor can affect the coefficients of insurance and wage-income variables. Yet, from the standpoint of policy, this bias may not be consequential. Without a fee variable, insurance influences both gross price—the fee charged—and net price—the price to the patient net of third-party payments. With a fee variable, the insurance variable's parameter would only incorporate the latter influence.

Private insurance coverage is represented by the variables FCOV, which takes the value one if the respondent is fully covered for visits to a doctor's office, and PCOV, which has the value of one if the respondent has partial coverage for these services. One may infer from the survey results (not presented) that persons with full coverage are generally affiliated with an independent plan, such as a union-sponsored group or prepaid group practice. Persons with partial coverage have a regular medical and/or a major medical plan.

Public insurance variables are VACOV for Veterans Administration coverage, MCAID for Medicaid (or Public Aid), and for the retiree group, MCARE for Medicare Part B. As we have defined the variables, a respondent may have both VA coverage and private insurance, but may not have private insurance and Medicaid concurrently. MCAID, FCOV, and PCOV are considered to be mutually exclusive. The MCAID variable has been eliminated from all but the female household head regressions because of the paucity of Medicaid recipients in the other three samples.

Time Price and Nonearned Income

As indicated in chapter 1, the shadow wage provides a measure of the value of a person's time. This wage may or may not be a fully valid indication of the value of time spent in obtaining ambulatory care. If time thus spent is personally distasteful, the shadow wage will understate the unit cost of patient time. If the patient enjoys going to the doctor, the shadow wage will overstate the unit cost of patient time. We do not have estimates of the intangible benefits that respondents get out of seeing the physician, but certainly our failure to measure this factor explicitly is unlikely to distort the analysis in any meaningful way.

There is reason to expect, as was noted in chapter 1, that job loss causes the shadow wage to fall. As a result, it is reasonable to hypothesize that the unemployed are less adverse to long waits in doctor's offices and hence are more likely to use hospital-based providers where waits are longer on the average.

For employed persons, the shadow wage equals the market wage, but the shadow wage exceeds the market wage for the nonemployed. Thus, the market wage is likely to be a good surrogate in one case, but not in the other. Shadow wages can in principal be derived for both kinds of individuals from an estimated labor supply function. Wages obtained in this way are conditional on: (1) work hours; (2) levels of "other" labor supply variables, such as nonearned income, age, sex, and marital status; and (3) the parameters of the labor supply function. One may assume work hours to be zero for purposes of projecting the shadow wage of unemployed persons; or, if one desires to account for time spent in job search, one may assume work hours to be at some low value.[23]

We have specified and estimated labor supply functions using MAS data expressly for the purpose of obtaining estimates of shadow wages. Unfortunately, although the estimated labor supply functions are reliable, gauged in terms of R^2s and t-values of the coefficients, the variance in the predicted shadow wages is unacceptably high. At zero work hours, we obtain predicted wages of a few cents while at forty work hours, shadow wages are $30 per hour and sometimes more.[24] The interested reader should consult the appendix for further details.

Rather than rely on implausible predictions, we have approximated the shadow wages in the following ways. For employed persons, the market hourly wage (HDY for household heads and *SPY* for spouses) represents the shadow wage. These market wages are predicted from a wage-generating equation and based on samples of working adults. This equation includes such variables as years of schooling completed, work experience, race-ethnicity, community size, a health status measure (other than the ones used in the access regressions), and region. The market wage generating equations are also presented in the appendix.

Our specification of the wage component for the nonemployed, a group consisting of adults outside the labor force and the unemployed, is more complex. On theoretical grounds, it can be said that the shadow wage of such persons exceeds the market wage. If so, the wage component may be specified as

$$\text{shadow wage} = \text{HDY} \cdot (1 + \Theta_1 D) \text{ for nonemployed heads} \qquad (5.1)$$

$$\text{shadow wage} = \text{SPY} \cdot (1 + \Theta_2 D) \text{ for nonemployed spouses,} \qquad (5.2)$$

where $D = 1$ for nonemployed and otherwise $= 0$.

If HDY and SPY consistently understate the shadow wages of nonemployed adults, Θ_i will be positive. However, we cannot rule out the possibility that nonemployed persons do not have the earnings potential of their employed counterparts. If so, the shadow wage of the nonemployed may in fact be lower than the market wages of employed persons on average; a negative Θ_i would reflect this. In the regressions presented in this and the following chapter, $HDY \cdot D$ = HEM and $SPY \cdot D$ = SEM for unemployed heads and spouses, respectively. Otherwise, HEM = SEM = 0.

To gauge the "pure" income effect on provider choice, two nonearned income variables have been specified: a measure of "permanent" nonearned family income (NEYP); and a measure of "unexplained" family income (RESID). The NEYP measure, discussed at length in the appendix, includes family income from interest and dividends, rents, Social Security retirement, private pensions, alimony or child support, armed forces allotment, and Veteran's Administration benefits. In constructing NEYP, we have assumed that families can count on income from these sources over the long term. The RESID measure includes income from "transitory" sources identified by the MAS: friends or relatives; unemployment compensation, Workman's Compensation; and public aid (welfare). In addition, the RESID measure includes some income remaining after subtracting (a) the predicted wages of the household head and spouse, (b) NEYP, and (c) the first component of RESID from actual family income ("explained transitory income"). Thus, as defined, RESID contains explained transitory income *and* unexplained family income; it may be positive or negative. Holding HDY, SPY, and NEYP constant, a family can be considered to be "lucky" if RESID is positive and "unlucky" if it is negative. By design, RESID represents unanticipated income; however, the possibility that it includes permanent elements (because it includes unexplained family income) cannot be ruled out. Specification of two nonearned income variables permits us, at least in principle, to assess asymmetries in responses to changes in permanent and transitory income.

Family Size

The influence of family size is represented by FSIZ. Since virtually all of our retiree families consist of two members, FSIZ is omitted from the retirees' regressions. As noted above, retirees living alone are excluded.

Race-Ethnicity

Race-ethnicity variables are BLACK and SURNAME, which equal one if the household head is black or Spanish-surnamed, respectively. SURNAME has been eliminated from regressions in which the proportion of Spanish-surnamed households was too small to permit us to derive reliable parameter estimates for the variable.

Reason for Visit

The MAS asked the respondents to describe the reasons for their visits and their responses were subsequently given numerical codes by the CHAS staff. Each reason was classified as being acute, chronic, or "other," and further classified by severity on a scale from one to four with four being the most severe.

We have defined five reasons for visit dummy variables: ASEV1 for acute visits of severity one and two; ASEV2 for acute visits of severity three and four; CSEV1 for chronic visits of severity one and two; CSEV2 for chronic visits of severity three and four; and CHKUP for visits in which the patient has no specific symptoms or visits made without reference to a specific chronic disease. To develop a mutually exclusive set of health variables, we have given priority to acute reasons over chronic over CHKUP. The acute diagnosis is more likely to be the primary reason for seeing the physician on a given date. Within acute and chronic codes, greater severity received priority over lesser severity. Thus each respondent was first screened for an ASEV2, then ASEV1, then a CSEV2, a CSEV1, and finally a CHKUP in descending priority.

Physician Availability

The final set of explanatory variables are physician-population ratios. The provider choice regressions contain variables representing office-based general practitioners and specialists per 10,000 population (GPPC and SPPC) and patient-care, hospital-based physicians per 10,000 population (HOSPC). All physician availability variables are defined for the respondent's Primary Sampling Unit (*PSU*). For metropolitan areas, a *PSU* is a county or a cluster of counties; for nonmetropolitan areas, *PSU*s are single counties.

Statistical Considerations and Estimation

Discriminant analysis is a form of multivariate analysis that is appropriately employed when the dependent variable identifies alternative groups or choices.[25] Functions are estimated which best distinguish among populations belonging to the respective groups. One of the most important uses of discriminant analysis is classification. Given an individual's characteristics and the estimated coefficients, classification scores are derived by multiplying classification coefficients by the values of the characteristics and adding. There is a vector of estimated coefficients for *each* of the alternatives, and the individual is classified as belonging to the alternative having the highest score. The estimated functions also have meaning in their own right. For example, if for three alternatives, the classification coefficients corresponding to the explanatory variable BLACK are 1.0,

2.2, and 3.3, respectively, blacks will be assigned to the third group, holding other factors constant (since $1.0 \cdot 1 = 1.0$, $2.2 \cdot 1 = 2.2$, and $3.3 \cdot 1 = 3.3$ when BLACK = 1). In many instances, the classification coefficients are negative, and the results also have meaning in such cases. For example, if the coefficients on BLACK were -1.0, -2.2, and -0.5, blacks would be assigned to the third category since being black subtracts least from the (total) score of the third group; in other words, the relative rather than the absolute values of the coefficients are the determining factor in classification.

Partial F-tests indicate the significance of the contribution of a specific characteristic, or equivalently explanatory variable to intergroup discrimination. Since the numerator degrees of freedom is one and the denominator degrees-of-freedom are large, the critical values of F for significance at 5 and one percent levels are 3.84 and 6.61.[26] Since the F follows the square of t when there is one degree-of-freedom in the numerator, $F = 1.0$ has about the same meaning as $t = 1.0$ in regression; t-values of 1.0 and greater are often taken as "suggestive" of an underlying relationship since explanatory variables with t's of 1.0 and above make positive contributions to corrected R^2s.

Our empirical results are evaluated in terms of the means and standard deviations associated with each of the provider groups, the classification function obtained from the discriminant analysis itself, and estimated probabilities that are based on the estimated classification function parameters. The means and standard deviations (included in parenthesis under the respective means in the following tables) and associated F-tests for significant differences among the means of the provider groups are useful for making bivariate (or two-way) comparisons among the groups. These results parallel the two-way contingency tables found in earlier chapters of this study. Bivariate comparisons are useful for drawing preliminary inferences about the nature of the population making specific choices. One might learn, for example, that the poor, blacks, and adults without private insurance tend to select institution-based physicians. However, although such comparisons permit one to isolate a cluster of explanatory variables that appear to be important, they do not permit one to isolate the individual contribution of each explanatory factor the the patient's decision about site of care. Discriminant analysis, as a multivariate technique, may be used for this purpose.

Our use of discriminant analysis as a basis for generating conditional probabilities is somewhat unusual, and the reader should be forewarned at the outset. This is common practice, however, with logit analysis. Economists often use discriminant analysis to derive starting values for logit analysis. In our experience with many logit regressions, the initial discriminant analysis estimates tend to be extremely close to final logit estimates. Thus we have taken the liberty of using the classification functions from discriminant analysis to derive predicted probabilities using the logit transform. The alternative with the highest predicted probability is also the group with the highest classification score in discriminant analysis. Readers who (because of their training in classical statistics) feel uncomfortable about our use of the logit transform may want to emphasize the effects of particular explanatory variables in classification rather than on the predicted probabilities.[27]

Empirical Results

The empirical results of our discriminant analysis of patient choice of provider are presented in tables 5-1 through 5-4. The retiree and female head results are easier to interpret because there are three rather than four alternatives and there are fewer explanatory variables. Therefore we begin our discussion of the provider choice results with these categories.

Retiree Results

Judging from the means and associated F-ratios, the primary differences among retirees selecting each of the three provider groups are in terms of physician availability and income. In particular, there is a close correspondence between patients choosing office-based specialists and the office-based specialist population ratio in the patient's Primary Sampling Unit (*PSU*). The means suggest that persons visiting GPs tend to live in areas with lower office-based specialist-population ratios.

    Differences in permanent (NEYP) and residual nonearned income (RESID) are also pronounced; patients of office-based specialists tend to be comparatively affluent. The patients of general practitioners rank second in terms of NEYP, but if RESID is added to NEYP, the patients of GPs have lower incomes than do the patients of institutional providers.

    Judging from the means on the left side of table 5-1, retired blacks and those without Medicare Part B constitute lower proportions of specialist physicians' patients,[28] but the group differences in these mean proportions are insignificant. Somewhat surprisingly, the Fs associated with the reason for visit proportions are uniformly small.

    Classification functions are presented on the right side of table 5-1. By and large, they confirm patterns evident from the means. Physician-population ratios are most helpful in distinguishing between office-based specialists' patients and patients of the other two provider types. Retirees with higher permanent nonearned income are more likely to see office-based specialists. The significance level of the RESID income variables is far lower, although there is an indication that retirees with higher levels of this type of income also have a higher likelihood of seeing office-based specialists. In fact, differences among the estimated RESID coefficients are greater than those for NEYP. The minor acute illness variable (ASEV1) is now statistically significant; judging from the classification coefficients associated with ASEV1, it is clear that the major difference is again between office-specialists' patients and patients choosing the other two alternatives. An *F*-test on differences among the estimated functions (take as a whole) reveals significant differences between the specialist patients and the two others, but not between patients of GPs and hospital-based providers. This test implies that retirees who see GPs are really not very different from those who see hospital-based physicians.

The estimated classification functions assign 62 percent of the retiree observations to the correct provider groups. If assignments had been made randomly, only 33 percent would have been correctly classified. The model is slightly more successful in classifying patients of office-based specialists; 66 percent of such patients are placed in the proper category versus 59 and 57 percent for the GP and hospital provider categories, respectively. Discriminant analysis enables us to classify the provider choices of retirees about twice as well as would assigning observations to provider types on a random basis.

Female Household Head Results

The means in table 5-2 suggest these patterns. There is an association between patient choice of provider and physician availability. Medicaid recipients comprise a substantially higher proportion of the female household head population that visit hospital-based physicians. Higher fractions of the patients of office-based specialists have private insurance covering their visits; and fewer of them are blacks and Spanish-surnamed patients. Hospital-based physicians have the highest fraction of both of these minorities. Hospital physicians also see higher proportions of female heads from large families.

Differences among the HDY and HEM means are statistically significant at conventional levels while those for NEYP and RESID are not, although in the case of NEYP, mean incomes of clinic patients are substantially lower. One may divide HEM by HDY to derive the proportions of nonworkers visiting each provider type. The proportions are 0.31, 0.11, and 0.38, respectively. As the underlying theory would predict, nonemployed persons are more likely to select time-intensive forms of care. Similarly, the mean wage rates of patients of office-based specialists are highest and those of the patients of clinics are lowest. As noted previously, the market wage equals the shadow wage for employed workers.

Although there are differences in proportions by reason for visit, only the minor acute illness variable (ASEV1) demonstrates statistically significant differences; office-based specialists have the lowest proportion of these patients.

Two sets of classification functions are presented in table 5-2, one with and one without the HEM variable. Including HEM improves the equation's

Table 5-1
Patient Choice of Provider: Retirees

Variable	Means and Standard Deviations ( )				Classification Coefficients			
	General Practitioner Office	Specialist Office	Outpatient-Emergency Room	$F_{(2,117)}$	General Practitioner Office	Specialist Office	Outpatient-Emergency Room	$F_{(1,107)}$
MDPC	8.69 (—)	11.25 (—)	9.89 (—)	—	—	—	—	—
GPPC	2.40 (0.87)	1.99 (0.63)	2.49 (1.15)	4.0†	4.41	3.57	4.73	5.2*
SPPC	1.15 (2.67)	6.06 (2.01)	4.57 (2.57)	8.3*	0.66	1.07	0.68	5.0*
HOSPC	2.14 (2.68)	3.20 (2.48)	2.83 (2.77)	2.2	0.21	0.07	0.36	1.4
PARTB	0.75 (0.44)	0.87 (0.20)	0.79 (0.43)	1.3	6.04	6.81	6.54	0.8
BLACK	0.12 (0.33)	0.06 (0.25)	0.21 (0.43)	1.3	3.33	3.48	4.62	0.7
NEYP	6334. (2482.)	7836. (2920.)	5937. (2368.)	5.2*	0.00068	0.00094	0.00065	4.9*
RESID	-776. (3153.)	984. (4015.)	-154. (3573.)	3.2†	0.00003	0.0002	0.00008	1.2
ASEV1	0.12 (0.33)	0.04 (0.20)	0.14 (0.36)	1.2	10.70	7.93	11.11	3.6*
ASEV2	0.05 (0.22)	0.09 (0.28)	0.21 (0.43)	2.0	12.21	12.10	14.95	1.6
CSEV1	0.53 (0.50)	0.53 (0.50)	0.43 (0.51)	0.2	9.69	8.58	9.82	1.1
CSEV2	0.09 (0.29)	0.19 (0.39)	0.07 (0.26)	—	—	—	—	—

CHKUP	0.22 (0.42)	0.15 (0.36)	0.14 (0.36)	0.5	10.29	8.61	10.16	1.6
CONSTANT	(−)	(−)	(−)	—	−16.12	−17.33	−18.15	—
Percent in group	49.2	39.2	11.7	—	—	—	—	—
Percent correctly classified	—	—	—	—	59.3	66.0	57.1	—

*Significant at 1 percent level; †significant at 5 percent level.

Table 5-2
Patient Choice of Provider: Female Heads

Variable	Means and Standard Deviations ( )				Classification Coefficients				Classification Coefficients			
	General Practitioner Office	Specialist Office	Outpatient-Emergency Room	$F_{(2,301)}$	General Practitioner Office	Specialist Office	Outpatient-Emergency Room	$F_{(1,286)}$	General Practitioner Office	Specialist Office	Outpatient-Emergency Room	$F_{(1,285)}$
MDPC	10.93 (—)	11.64 (—)	12.01 (—)	—	—	—	—	—	—	—	—	—
GPPC	2.31 (0.99)	2.04 (0.92)	1.92 (0.59)	4.5†	3.28	2.82	2.94	4.2†	3.28	2.83	2.94	4.0†
SPPC	5.57 (2.67)	6.18 (1.04)	5.78 (2.46)	2.1	1.17	1.31	1.06	3.4	1.17	1.30	1.06	3.0
HOSPC	3.05 (2.63)	3.42 (2.51)	4.31 (2.87)	4.2†	0.09	0.00	0.33	6.0†	0.09	0.01	0.33	5.6*
MCAID	0.24 (0.43)	0.06 (0.24)	0.33 (0.48)	11.4*	0.67	-0.14	1.16	3.0	0.80	0.31	1.05	0.9
FCOV	0.02 (0.14)	0.09 (0.28)	0.08 (0.28)	3.0†	-0.80	0.52	0.33	2.4	-0.85	0.35	0.37	2.2
PCOV	0.20 (0.40)	0.32 (0.47)	0.15 (0.36)	4.0†	1.69	2.30	1.51	2.0	1.62	2.08	1.56	0.9
BLACK	0.23 (0.42)	0.18 (0.39)	0.35 (0.48)	2.8	3.69	2.87	4.00	3.3	3.69	2.87	4.00	3.2
SURNAME	0.15 (0.36)	0.03 (0.18)	0.17 (0.38)	5.4*	0.92	0.03	1.00	1.7	0.93	0.06	1.00	1.6
FSIZ	2.39 (1.73)	1.90 (1.47)	2.79 (1.74)	5.8*	1.28	1.31	1.39	0.3	1.27	1.27	1.40	0.5
NEYP	1897. (2221.)	1855. (1707.)	1187. (1559.)	2.6	0.0005	0.0004	0.0004	1.3	0.0005	0.0005	0.0003	1.2

	(1)	(2)	(3)	(4)	(5)	(6)	(7)	(8)	(9)	(10)	(11)	(12)
RESID	-16.5 (4861.)	-198. (4688.)	14.2 (3900.)	0.1	0.0001	0.0001	0.0001	0.2	0.0001	0.0001	0.0000	1.5
HDY	4.58 (1.49)	4.90 (1.69)	4.24 (1.58)	3.2†	2.09	2.14	2.01	0.5	2.11	2.19	1.99	1.0
HEM	1.42 (2.15)	0.55 (1.61)	1.62 (2.16)	8.1*	–	–	–	–	-0.08	0.27	0.06	4.3†
ASEV1	0.18 (0.38)	0.08 (0.27)	0.19 (0.39)	3.1†	15.1	14.5	15.8	1.2	15.1	14.5	15.8	1.1
ASEV2	0.13 (0.33)	0.22 (0.41)	0.21 (0.41)	2.0	13.4	13.8	14.5	1.1	13.4	13.8	14.5	1.1
CSEV1	0.45 (0.50)	0.33 (0.47)	0.31 (0.47)	2.4	15.0	14.7	15.1	0.1	15.0	14.8	15.1	0.1
CSEV2	0.09 (0.29)	0.10 (0.31)	0.02 (0.14)	–	–	–	–	–	–	–	–	–
CHKUP	0.16 (0.36)	0.27 (0.45)	0.27 (0.45)	2.9	13.1	13.7	14.4	1.7	13.1	13.8	14.4	1.6
CONSTANT	– (–)	– (–)	– (–)	–	-21.2	-20.7	-21.4	–	-21.2	-20.8	-21.4	–
Percent in group	46.4	37.8	15.8	–	–	–	–	–	–	–	–	–
Percent correctly classified	–	–	–	–	44.0	63.5	56.2	–	41.8	68.7	56.2	–

*Significant at 1 percent level; †significant at 5 percent level.

predictive ability slightly. Fifty-three percent of the observations are classified correctly when HEM is not included and 54 percent when HEM is included. Moreover, the variable is statistically significant at the 5 percent level when included. Thus we shall emphasize the second set of estimated functions.

In contrast to the means, few explanatory variables attain statistical significance. To a considerable extent, the decline in significant variables reflects multicollinearity. The reader will recall that the partial Fs reflect the *additional* contribution of a particular variable to discrimination, given the other included explanatory variables. If much of the influence has already been represented, most likely the variable will be insignificant. This would seem to be the case in the context of the MCAID variable; it is almost statistically significant before HEM is included; but with HEM, the F falls to a value below one.

The physician-population variables are defined for *PSU*s and are therefore less closely related to the other explanatory variables which relate to characteristics of individual patients. Two of the three physician-population variables are statistically significant at the 5 percent level or better. The associated coefficients are plausible and indicate rather clearly that physician availability affects patient choice of provider type.

One must be cautious when drawing inferences about the effects of third-party reimbursement from table 5-2. The coefficients indicate that Medicaid female household heads have a higher propensity to select clinics, and those with private insurance are more likely to go to office-based specialists. However, the associated Fs are not high, especially with HEM in the equation. We shall discuss this matter further when we assess the predicted probabilities, based on the coefficients in table 5-2.

Race proved to be unimportant in the case of retirees, but the variable BLACK is almost significant at the 5 percent level in the case of female heads. The partial F associated with SURNAME is lower, but like BLACK, the coefficients imply that female heads in this minority group are more likely to visit physicians in institutional settings. Unfortunately, the results presented in table 5-2 do not allow us to distinguish between two alternative hypotheses, namely: Office-based physicians discriminate against minorities; or, minorities choose clinics because they work and live in close proximity to the location of clinics.

Overall, the wage-income variables clearly imply that the choices of provider by female household heads reflect ability to pay. All classification function coefficients point to this, although one must add that most of the Fs indicate levels of significance below 0.05. Among the time price-income variables, HEM is the best discriminating variable by far. As we have noted, for nonemployed workers, the shadow wage exceeds the market wage. In some cases, nonworkers have relatively high shadow wages; in others, the market wage is comparatively low (that is, lower than the wage of workers with many of the same characteristics). Recessions reduce the market wage offered many individuals. If the high shadow wage person dominated the female heads' sample, one would expect to observe that nonemployed heads use time-intensive sources of care less frequently on the average, not more often. Thus it is reasonable to infer that the low shadow wage person dominates the sample. Nonemployed females face lower wages on the average than those predicted by our wage-generating regression that is based on observations of employed persons. A transitory income loss effect may also play a role in provider choice. The RESID variable incorporates some income from identifiable transitory sources as well as unexplained family income. Judging from the classification coefficients associated with RESID, it is evident that this variable has only very small impact on provider choice.

One might infer from the data in table 5-2 that decreased work opportunities resulting from a recession lead to greater reliance on hospital sources of ambulatory care, but no evidence on lag structure can be gleaned from these data. We do not know how long a female head would have to be out of the work force before provider choice would be affected. Nonearned income plays a role, but we cannot say how long it would take for a policy of increased transfer payments to have an impact on choice of practice setting.

The reason for visit variables prove to be unimportant overall in this case as they were in the case of retirees. We cannot rule out the possibility that more detailed diagnostic mix variables might have produced a better result. But for the present, it is reasonable to conclude that reason for visits is not an important determinant, especially in comparison to physician availability and patient socioeconomic status.

The overall predictive ability of the female head discriminant regressions is lower than that for retirees. The model is least satisfactory in predicting which female heads visit office-based general practitioners. While the estimated functions only classify 42 percent of the general practitioner observations correctly, they are on target 69 and 56 percent of the time, respectively, in assigning observations to the office-based specialist and hospital-based categories.

Married Male Results

The married male results, reported in table 5-3, reinforce some of the earlier results, but also relate important differences. Some of the differences undoubtedly reflect the fact that outpatient clinics are distinguished from emergency room visits. This is probably a major factor in the more pronounced differences among the provider types in terms of reason for visit than were evident in either of the two preceding tables.

As above, there are statistically significant differences in the means of the physician availability variables. The patterns of the GPPC and SPPC means are plausible, but those associated with HOSPC require further discussion. For the first time, emergency room visits are considered separately. As one can tell from a simple comparison of the means for MDPC, which represents the sum of GPPC,

Table 5-3
Patient Choice of Provider: Married Males

Variable	Means and Standard Deviations ( )					Classification Coefficients				
	General Practitioner Office	Specialist Office	Outpatient Department	Emergency Room	$F_{(3,506)}$	General Practitioner Office	Specialist Office	Outpatient Department	Emergency Room	$F_{(1,491)}$
MDPC	9.75 (—)	11.04 (—)	10.75 (—)	9.15 (—)	—	—	—	—	—	—
GPPC	2.39 (1.05)	2.08 (0.69)	2.01 (0.69)	2.18 (0.64)	5.4*	4.64	4.42	4.25	4.43	2.05
SPPC	4.69 (2.32)	5.52 (2.07)	5.48 (2.19)	5.03 (2.28)	5.3*	1.43	1.56	1.51	1.71	2.10
HOSPC	2.67 (2.61)	3.44 (2.72)	3.26 (2.58)	1.94 (2.09)	4.0*	-0.19	-0.17	-0.17	-0.48	2.02
FCOV	0.06 (0.23)	0.11 (0.31)	0.07 (0.25)	0.14 (0.36)	1.7	-0.29	1.07	0.14	1.54	1.63
PCOV	0.43 (0.50)	0.50 (0.50)	0.36 (0.48)	0.29 (0.46)	2.0	-0.47	-0.18	-0.79	-0.64	1.15
VACOV	0.06 (0.23)	0.06 (0.23)	0.15 (0.36)	0.10 (0.30)	2.6	-0.04	-0.36	1.31	0.63	2.40
BLACK	0.08 (0.27)	0.07 (0.26)	0.10 (0.30)	0.14 (0.36)	0.6	3.29	3.35	3.53	3.71	0.12
SURNAME	0.10 (0.30)	0.04 (0.19)	0.12 (0.33)	0.05 (0.22)	2.2	-0.67	-1.15	0.24	-2.09	2.25
FSIZ	3.68 (1.49)	3.54 (1.31)	3.63 (1.66)	4.05 (1.94)	0.8	2.13	2.12	2.10	2.26	0.24
NEYP	715. (2387.)	1790. (2836.)	1166. (2802.)	329. (2083.)	6.2*	0.0002	0.0004	0.0003	0.0002	4.35†
RESID	-381. (6119.)	318. (6111.)	-960. (6005.)	-1825. (5787.)	1.7	0.0001	0.0001	0.0001	0.0001	1.78

HDY	6.87 (2.00)	7.46 (2.18)	7.14 (2.39)	5.92 (2.10)	4.5*	1.58	1.66	1.69	1.36	1.88
HEM	0.53 (1.89)	0.60 (2.07)	0.61 (2.08)	0.13 (0.61)	0.4	—	—	—	—	—
SPY	4.59 (1.72)	4.58 (1.59)	4.27 (1.79)	3.95 (1.26)	1.7	1.19	1.08	0.95	1.11	1.87
SEM	2.35 (2.56)	2.47 (2.54)	2.15 (2.38)	1.63 (2.21)	0.8	—	—	—	—	—
ASEV1	0.29 (0.45)	0.15 (0.36)	0.19 (0.39)	0.52 (0.51)	6.9*	41.98	41.19	40.91	43.92	1.22
ASEV2	0.19 (0.40)	0.28 (0.45)	0.19 (0.39)	0.24 (0.44)	1.4	41.77	42.04	41.20	42.67	0.29
CSEV1	0.31 (0.46)	0.38 (0.49)	0.29 (0.46)	0.24 (0.44)	1.0	41.97	42.07	41.32	42.64	0.23
CSEV2	0.02 (0.02)	0.03 (0.03)	0.03 (0.03)	0.00 (0.00)	—	—	—	—	—	—
CHKUP	0.19 (0.39)	0.17 (0.38)	0.31 (0.46)	0.00 (0.00)	3.5†	40.70	40.34	40.88	40.38	0.11
CONSTANT	— (−)	— (−)	— (−)	— (−)	—	−41.21	−41.71	−40.13	−41.36	—
Percent in group	56.7	27.6	11.6	4.1	—	—	—	—	—	—
Percent correctly classified	—	—	—	—	—	34.3	49.6	50.8	81.0	—

*Significant at 1 percent level; †significant at 5 percent level.

SPPC, and HOSPC, the patient-care physician-population ratio is lowest in the emergency room category. As noted in previous literature, individuals often use emergency rooms for nonemergency care because physicians are unavailable in other settings, not because emergency rooms are well staffed. Thus, the low mean value of HOSPC, corresponding to men who saw physicians in emergency rooms, is not surprising. We are not able to explain the fact that the mean for HOSPC associated with the outpatient department category is less than that for the office-based specialist category.

There are significant differences in the means of permanent nonearned income of the family (NEYP) and the market wage for the male head (HDY). In both cases, patients of office-based specialists have the highest value and emergency room patients have the lowest value. The RESID variable exhibits a similar pattern, but the differences in means are not statistically significant at conventional levels. With the exception of RESID, incomes are higher for the third than for the first provider type, a result seemingly inconsistent with the results for retirees and female heads outlined above. Again, the differences are in large part attributable to the four-way as opposed to the three-way categorization in earlier tables. Some visits to clinics represent referrals from office-based physicians and there is no reason to expect such patients to have relatively low incomes.

Mean potential market wages of female spouses (SPY) are higher for husbands who are patients of office-based physicians. If household time of husband and spouse are substitutes, an increase in the wife's wage would induce the husband to allocate a greater proportion of his time to household activities and time-intensive consumption, holding other factors, including the "pure" income effect, constant. The income effect associated with an increase in the wife's wage, however, may induce the husband to spend less time in market work; but, at the same time, both husband and wife would engage in less time-intensive consumption. The observed pattern in the means of SPY suggest that the latter force dominates.

Neither the HEM nor the SEM variable, however, exhibit any variation in means according to provider type. A higher proportion of married male emergency room patients are employed (0.98) than is the case for patients in the other three categories (0.92, 0.92, and 0.91, respectively). The proportions for the female heads, by contrast, were substantially different.

The estimated classification functions assign 42 percent of the married male observations to the correct provider types, as compared to 25 percent correct assignments if the observations were assigned randomly. The model predicts emergency room patients quite well (81 percent of observations assigned correctly), but its ability to predict patients of office-based general practitioners is poor (34 percent, correctly).

The classification functions are generally consistent with the patterns in the variable means. Although only one variable, NEYP, attains statistical significance at conventional levels, partial *F*s corresponding to several variables, physician availability (GPPC, SPPC, HOSPC), Veteran's Administration coverage (VACOV) and Spanish-surnamed persons (SURNAME), exceed two. In contrast to female heads, race, as judged by the performance of BLACK, plays no role in choice of provider. On the other hand, the pattern for SURNAME is roughly similar to the pattern exhibited in the case of female heads.

Married Females

Provider choice results for married females are presented in table 5–4. A high proportion of the differences among variable means are significant at the 5 percent level or higher. Differences in physician availability means are all significant; patterns in HOSPC reinforce our findings for married men. But unlike the findings for married men, differences among partial insurance (PCOV) means are significant at the 5 percent level. The pattern among the means, however, is similar to that for men. Patients of office-based specialists and emergency room patients are the most and least likely, respectively, to be partially covered by a private insurer.

As in the cases of retirees and married men, there are no significant differences in the fractions of black patients by provider type. Differences in the surname proportions are significant and in this respect parallel the female head results more closely. Family size (FSIZ) differences are insignificant as they were in the case of married males. Even in the case of female heads where FSIZ differences in means were significant, the variable had no discernible impact in the discriminant analysis.

There are obvious similarities in the patterns of the wage-income variables for married women and the results for these variables presented in earlier tables. The relative values of the NEYP, RESID, and HDY means are similar. But HDY requires a different interpretation in this context since we are now examining wives' rather than husbands' use of physicians' services. The results do *not* suggest that wives are more likely to engage in time-intensive consumption when husbands earn more. Quite the contrary. Both wife and husband tend to utilize sources of care that are less costly in terms of patient time. The provider type decision, of course, involves more than patient time considerations; for a combination of reasons, more affluent households purchase office-based specialist care on the average.

The usefulness of distinguishing among households according to family structure becomes quite evident when one examines patterns in SPY and SEM. First, if one divides SEM by SPY, one obtains the fractions of married women in the sample who are not employed. These fractions are 0.48, 0.56, 0.49, and 0.26 for the four provider categories. In contrast to nonemployed female heads who were least likely to visit office-based specialists, female spouses are most

Table 5-4
Patient Choice of Provider: Married Females

Variable	Means and Standard Deviations					Classification Coefficients									
	General Practitioner Office	Specialist Office	Outpatient Department	Emergency Room	$F_{(3,599)}$	General Practitioner Office	Specialist Office	Outpatient Department	Emergency Room	$F_{(1,586)}$	General Practitioner Office	Specialist Office	Outpatient Department	Emergency Room	$F_{(1,584)}$
MDPC	9.68 (−)	11.64 (−)	9.38 (−)	7.71 (−)	−	−	−	−	−	−	−	−	−	−	−
GPPC	2.40 (0.90)	2.16 (0.89)	2.01 (0.58)	2.00 (0.71)	5.3*	4.17	3.99	3.60	3.42	3.95†	4.19	4.02	3.60	3.39	4.27†
SPPC	4.75 (2.54)	5.90 (1.99)	4.76 (2.36)	4.08 (2.44)	13.0*	1.29	1.47	1.23	1.19	4.80†	1.31	1.50	1.24	1.17	5.14†
HOSPC	2.53 (2.60)	3.57 (2.73)	2.61 (2.41)	1.63 (2.02)	8.7*	−0.43	−0.43	−0.46	−0.55	0.25	−0.44	−0.44	−0.46	−0.53	0.13
FCOV	0.04 (0.20)	0.06 (0.25)	0.13 (0.33)	0.07 (0.26)	1.6	−0.76	−0.44	0.91	−0.08	1.53	−0.67	−0.33	0.97	−0.13	1.44
PCOV	0.37 (0.48)	0.47 (0.50)	0.30 (0.46)	0.27 (0.46)	2.9†	0.32	0.65	0.19	0.17	1.21	0.33	0.64	0.28	0.30	0.93
BLACK	0.09 (0.29)	0.09 (0.28)	0.18 (0.38)	0.13 (0.35)	1.2	5.48	5.40	6.43	5.55	0.86	5.66	5.61	6.58	5.50	0.77
SURNAME	0.13 (0.34)	0.06 (0.24)	0.10 (0.30)	0.20 (0.41)	2.9†	1.47	0.77	1.76	2.56	2.30	1.51	0.80	1.83	2.59	2.29
FSIZ	4.03 (1.52)	3.87 (1.48)	3.92 (1.86)	3.60 (1.50)	0.8	2.35	2.32	2.33	2.11	0.56	2.37	2.34	2.39	2.16	0.49
NEYP	449. (1997.)	1053. (2299.)	888. (2853.)	162. (2243.)	3.8*	−0.00011	−0.00001	0.00002	−0.00010	1.96	−0.00015	−0.00005	−0.00005	−0.00014	1.70
RESID	−769. (5966.)	355. (5958.)	−1548. (6002.)	−1272. (5285.)	2.3	−0.00002	0.00001	−0.00004	−0.00004	1.52	−0.00007	−0.00005	−0.00012	−0.00007	1.77
HDY	6.62 (2.06)	7.10 (2.37)	6.70 (2.46)	5.64 (1.76)	3.6†	1.34	1.34	1.39	1.14	0.64	1.34	1.35	1.38	1.12	0.71
HEM	0.35 (1.58)	0.29 (1.31)	0.93 (2.32)	0.91 (2.29)	2.5	−	−	−	−	−	0.18	0.14	0.48	0.45	3.24
SPY	4.40 (1.72)	4.54 (1.58)	4.35 (1.64)	4.43 (1.99)	0.4	1.37	1.31	1.26	1.50	0.63	1.27	1.20	1.16	1.50	1.07
SEM	2.09 (2.42)	2.56 (2.53)	2.15 (2.37)	1.15 (1.95)	2.8	−	−	−	−	−	0.27	0.30	0.33	0.07	1.21

ASEV1	0.22 (0.41)	0.08 (0.27)	0.03 (0.16)	0.07 (0.26)	9.4*	13.80	12.93	12.52	13.87	1.92	13.67	12.82	12.22	13.67	2.00
ASEV2	0.17 (0.38)	0.14 (0.35)	0.20 (0.41)	0.27 (0.46)	0.8	12.93	12.86	13.08	14.63	0.71	12.91	12.82	13.06	14.63	0.73
CSEV1	0.32 (0.47)	0.44 (0.50)	0.50 (0.51)	0.60 (0.51)	4.7	12.53	12.99	13.20	14.46	1.46	12.39	12.84	12.98	14.64	1.44
CSEV2	0.08 (0.08)	0.07 (0.07)	0.08 (0.08)	0.07 (0.07)	—	—	—	—	—	—	—	—	—	—	—
CHKUP	0.21 (0.41)	0.27 (0.45)	0.20 (0.41)	0.07 (0.26)	1.8	11.50	11.81	11.59	12.24	0.30	11.45	11.76	11.51	12.20	0.30
CON-STANT	— (−)	— (−)	— (−)	— (−)	—	−25.88	−26.39	−24.65	−23.55	—	−26.07	−26.61	−25.10	−23.77	—
Percent in group	49.9	40.9	6.6	2.5	—	—	—	—	—	—	—	—	—	—	—
Percent correctly classified	—	—	—	—	—	40.2	51.4	30.0	66.7	—	38.9	54.3	40.0	66.7	—

*Significant at 1 percent level; †significant at 5 percent level.

likely to do so. It is reasonable to conjecture that the motives for not working differ. For female heads, the reason tends to be inadequate employment opportunities; for married women, it is a comparatively high shadow wage—probably in large part a reflection of their husbands' high earnings. Second, there are no differences in potential market wages for the wife (SPY) by provider type. Income from other sources appears to be a far more reliable predictor.

There are several significant differences in the reason for visit proportions, but the patterns are not always consistent with those for married males. Apparent contradictions may reflect either biological differences between the sexes and/or anomalies in the method we used for classifying particular diagnoses as acute or chronic.

The two sets of discriminant functions assign married women to the correct provider category 43 and 45 percent of the time, a slightly better performance than in the case of married men. As with the married men, the model identifies emergency room patients best and is worst in identifying patients of office-based general practitioners.

Both office-based generalist- and specialist-populations ratio (GPPC and SPPC) variables have significant impacts on decisions at the 5 percent level, and the patterns in the coefficients themselves imply that physician availability matters. This has been a consistent result throughout this analysis. Availability of hospital-based physicians, however, demonstrates no effect.

Although there are significant differences in the PCOV means, the partial Fs associated with PCOV's classification coefficients are low, especially with the inclusion of the employment status variables HEM and SEM. This result also occurred in the discriminant analysis on the sample of female household heads. The NEYP and RESID results are broadly consistent with results reported above.

The HEM coefficients imply that wives of nonemployed husbands are more likely to utilize institutional sources of ambulatory care. Although this result is not surprising, it is somewhat surprising that table 5-3 did not reveal that nonemployed husbands also use these sources of care more often. The partial F associated with the HEM variable in a variant of the discriminant analysis of the male sample (not reported in table 5-3) was 0.5 versus 3.2 in table 5-4. These results imply that the wife rather than the husband faces reallocations as the result of the husband's job loss. Patterns in the SEM classification coefficients differ markedly from those of the HEM, but are similar to the patterns in SEM means discussed above.

Predicted Probabilities

Table 5-5, in which conditional predictions are presented, serves two purposes. First, it provides us with estimates of magnitudes of response. Second, it allows us to review certain key findings. The number of possible combinations of

Table 5-5
Predicted Probabilities

Variables	Retirees (3 Alternatives)							Female Heads (3 Alternatives)					Married Men (4 Alternatives)					Married Women (4 Alternatives)				
	R1	R2	R3	R4	R5	R6	R7	FH1	FH2	FH3	FH4	FH5	MM1	MM2	MM3	MM4	MM5	MW1	MW2	MW3	MW4	MW5
Assumptions																						
GPPC	M	M	M	M	3.0	M	M	M	M	M	M	3.0	M	M	M	M	3.0	M	M	M	M	3.0
SPPC	M	M	M	M	0.0	M	M	M	M	M	M	0.0	M	M	M	M	0.0	M	M	M	M	0.0
HOSPC	M	M	M	M	1.0	M	M	M	M	M	M	1.0	M	M	M	M	1.0	M	M	M	M	1.0
MCAID	—	—	—	—	—	—	—	—	—	—	—	—	—	—	—	—	—	—	—	—	—	—
FCOV	—	—	—	—	—	—	—	1	—	—	—	—	—	—	—	1	—	—	—	—	1	—
PCOV	—	—	—	—	—	—	—	—	—	—	—	—	—	—	1	—	—	—	—	1	—	—
PARTB	1	1	1	1	1	1	1	—	—	—	—	—	—	—	—	—	—	—	—	—	—	—
BLACK	1	1	1	—	—	1	1	—	—	—	—	—	—	—	—	—	—	—	—	—	—	—
SURNAME	0	0	0	0	0	0	0	0	0	0	0	0	0	0	0	0	0	0	0	0	0	0
FSIZ	4000	4000	7000	7000	7000	15000	25000	3.0	3.0	3.0	3.0	3.0	4.0	4.0	4.0	4.0	4.0	4.0	4.0	4.0	4.0	4.0
NEYP	0	0	0	7000	0	15000	25000	0	0	0	1000	0	0	0	2000	3000	0	0	0	2000	3000	0
RESID	—	—	—	—	—	—	—	2.30	2.30	2.30	10.00	2.30	2.30	2.30	20.00	30.00	2.30	2.30	2.30	20.00	30.00	2.30
HDY	—	—	—	—	—	—	—	—	—	—	—	—	—	—	—	—	—	—	—	—	—	—
HEM	—	—	—	—	—	—	—	—	—	—	—	—	2.30	2.30	2.30	2.30	2.30	2.30	2.30	2.30	2.30	2.30
SPY	—	—	—	—	—	—	—	—	—	—	—	—	—	—	—	—	—	—	—	—	—	—
SEM	0	0	0	0	0	0	0	0	0	0	0	0	0	0	0	0	0	0	0	0	0	0
ASEV1	0	0	0	0	0	0	0	0	0	0	0	0	0	0	0	0	0	0	0	0	0	0
ASEV2	1	1	1	1	1	1	1	1	1	1	1	1	1	1	1	1	1	1	1	1	1	1
CSEV1	0	0	0	0	0	0	0	0	0	0	0	0	0	0	0	0	0	0	0	0	0	0
CHKUP																						
Predictions																						
General Practitioner Office	0.23	0.45	0.18	0.38	0.43	0.08	0.01	0.27	0.28	0.26	0.26	0.64	0.52	0.59	0.42	0.18	0.68	0.18	0.20	0.23	0.25	0.27
Specialist Office	0.13	0.22	0.29	0.40	0.19	0.86	0.99	0.11	0.25	0.15	0.71	0.21	0.11	0.12	0.37	0.49	0.10	0.22	0.26	0.45	0.36	0.12
Outpatient-Emergency Room Combined	0.64	0.33	0.53	0.22	0.36	0.06	0.00	0.62	0.47	0.59	0.03	0.15	0.37	0.29	0.21	0.33	0.22	0.61	0.54	0.32	0.39	0.62
Outpatient Department	—	—	—	—	—	—	—	—	—	—	—	—	0.10	0.09	0.21	0.33	0.08	0.33	0.15	0.31	0.39	0.20
Emergency Room	—	—	—	—	—	—	—	—	—	—	—	—	0.27	0.20	0.00	0.00	0.14	0.28	0.39	0.01	0.00	0.41

assumed values of the explanatory variables is limitless; we have selected only a few of the more interesting ones. An *"M"* in table 5-5 indicates that the mean for the entire sample has been assumed for the purpose of generating the prediction. That is, unlike the means in tables 5-1 through 5-4, the means designated by *M* are identical for all three, or four, provider alternatives. There are several variants per demographic group: R1 through R7 for retirees; FH1 through FH5 for female household heads; MM1 through MM5 for married men; and MW1 through MW5 for married women. When two sets of classification functions were presented above, we have taken the second set for purposes of preparing table 5-5.

The impacts of changes in physician availability may be assessed by comparing variants R4 and R5, FH2, and FH5, MM2 and MM5, and MW2 and MW5. Each pair holds all variables except physician-population ratios constant. Our comparison is between a hypothetical community with sample mean values of the physician-population ratios and a community with three office-based general practitioners and one hospital-based physician per 10,000 population. Such an area is not "medically underserved" according to the value of one physician per 4,000 population that is often used by the Department of Health, Education, and Welfare as the standard for underserved areas, but it is far below the national average in terms of physician availability. As seen in table 5-5, physician-population ratios have powerful effects on the predicted probabilities. Office-based general practitioners always increase in relative importance and specialists always decrease in variance containing the low physician-population ratios. The impacts on the use of clinics and emergency rooms vary. Retirees and married women are more likely to use hospital sources of ambulatory care in low physician-population ratio areas; the opposite results hold for the other two samples. These latter results withstanding, a close association between physician availability and patient choice of provider is suggested by the results in table 5-5.

The sample sizes on the Medicaid variable only permitted us to include MCAID in the female head analysis. Although there were significant differences in the means, the partial Fs associated with the MCAID variables in the discriminant analysis were low. Variants FH2 and FH3 are identical except that FH2 assumes the female head is a Medicaid recipient; differences in predicted probabilities are quite small.

Private insurance coverage and income are varied jointly in table 5-5. Female head variants FH3 and FH4 allow us to compare an employed female head without private coverage for doctors' services, a market wage at the Federal minimum, and no income from nonemployment sources with an employed head with a $10 hourly wage (about $20,000 annual salary), and $1,000 annual permanent nonearned income, say from bonds. A FH3 female head is predicted to seek care from a hospital-based provider; the likelihood that her FH4 counterparts will do so is virtually nil. Similar results are obtained for retirees. In the case of married persons, the combination of private insurance coverage and higher wage and nonwage income leads to a move away from GPs and emergency rooms toward the other sources.

The predicted probabilities presented in table 5-5 also allow us to make comparisons of black-white provider choices. In light of the earlier results on race, which showed black-white differences to be most pronounced in the case of female heads, comparisons between the FH1 and FH2 variants merit most attention. In these cases, whites are far more likely to visit office-based specialists, holding other factors, including family income, constant.

Conclusions and Implications

In this chapter variations in one dimension of access have been investigated with a single 1975 cross-section. As noted at the outset of this chapter, the implications of this analysis concern not only the effects of economic conditions on access to ambulatory care, but the effects of more general health care policies, such as those related to health manpower, as well. Some of the inferences drawn from the empirical analysis are by necessity indirect and, unfortunately, as emphasized previously, no information about the response lags can be obtained from a single cross-section.

The retirees and female head regressions have been more informative on the whole than those for married persons aged 25 to 64. There are at least two reasons for the comparatively superior performance of the first two demographic groups. First, mean incomes of retirees and female-headed households are far lower than incomes of households with husband and wife present. It is plausible to expect that the effects of the financial variables are nonlinear, that is, important at low levels of wages and income with diminishing effects thereafter. To the extent that this is so, "average" impacts of adverse conditions in the economy for the population as a whole, like those reported estimates in chapter 3, may greatly understate the effects on the disadvantaged. Second, the models for married persons are more complex. We have attempted to capture the impacts of the husband's market opportunities on the wife's behavior and vice versa. The results in this respect are sometimes ambiguous, but some regressions suggest asymmetries. Thus, for example, the wife's use of physicians' services appears to be more affected by the husband's employment status than is that of the husband himself. Further research should explicitly consider these asymmetries.

Subject to these limitations, the research reported in this chapter has yielded a few important findings.

Our primary thrust in this and other chapters has been to attempt to gauge the impact of the 1974-1975 inflation-recession on patient access to physicians' services. To accomplish this objective, we developed specific wage and income variables. As discussed more fully in the appendix, we attempted to derive a measure of the patient's shadow wage. As work hours of the unemployed or underemployed fall, so does the person's shadow wage. As a consequence, such persons may be expected to be less averse to engaging in time-intensive activities. The method for obtaining shadow wages failed to yield plausible estimates. Thus, we have approximated the theoretically desired measure with market wages and the variables HEM and SEM, which allow for differential wage impacts for the nonemployed heads and spouses. Adult household members do not work for two basic reasons: the asking price of their labor is comparatively high; and/or the wage they currently are able to obtain in the market is comparatively low. The vast majority of men and large numbers of female heads are not employed for the second reason; a higher proportion of wives do not work for the first reason. Persons with relatively high shadow wages may be expected to select less time-intensive forms of medical care consumption.

We find that nonemployed female heads are more likely to utilize hospital-based sources of ambulatory care. Moreover, there is some indication that a husband's nonemployment leads his wife to select a hospital-based physician. No similar effect is apparent for husbands. That is, when husbands do not work, they do not tend to choose outpatient clinics or emergency rooms. Among the three samples for which the employment status applies, the female head results merit the most definite conclusions with regard to the effects of job loss. Caveats with respect to response lags withstanding, it seems likely that recessions increase the proportion of female heads using hospital-based physicians.

For employed persons, the market wage equals the shadow wage. Thus, as the market wage rises, we expect such individuals to attempt to reduce their own time input in consumption. High wage individuals are also wealthier. Their resources are in part allocated to purchasing various types of amenities, including the kinds of process variables considered in this and other chapters. Estimates of market wage impacts are again most reliable for female heads. As market wages rise, female heads tend to switch from hospital- to office-based sources of care. At least on the basis of our empirical results, we can be much less confident about the effects of labor market conditions on married persons.

We have also gauged the partial impacts of nonearned income on access. Variables NEYP and RESID represent permanent nonemployment income and transitory-residual income, respectively. The latter includes transfer payments, assumed to be transitory (unemployment compensation, public assistance), but it also incorporates unexplained income from other (unaccounted for) sources. We are very reluctant to draw any conclusions about the impacts on access of any particular type of nonemployment income. However, it can be stated that nonemployment income has anticipated impacts on access of retirees and female heads in particular. Our results establish a link, for example, between *real* Social Security benefits and retiree access. If such benefits were to fall in real terms as a consequence of inflation, retirees would eventually place greater reliance on the hospital-based physician.

Since most persons with private health insurance are covered by group policies provided by employers, there is a definite connection between loss of employment and private health insurance. Recent research by Sloan implies that private health insurance coverage affects choice of provider.[29] Our results on the partial effects of private insurance are weaker, but in the case of female heads and married males, there is some evidence that loss of private coverage affects the site of care.

Medicaid is an alternative to private insurance for the unemployed in particular and the disadvantaged in general. Recent work by Sloan, Cromwell, and Mitchell indicated that most office-based physicians are reluctant to accept large numbers of Medicaid patients, especially when Medicaid fee schedules are comparatively low and associated administrative burdens ("red tape") are high.[30] Medicaid effects have only been assessed in the analysis of female heads. We are unable to discern a partial Medicaid effect on provider choice in this area.

There is concern about patient access to physicians' services in general, but there is widespread agreement among policy makers that the problems of minorities, including blacks and Spanish-Americans, merit special attention. Our analysis points out instances when race-ethnicity affects patients' choices, but the effects of minority status are not uniform across samples, even qualitatively speaking.

Recent policy actions, among them the 1976 Health Professions Educational Assistance Act, have the objective of increasing the availability of primary care physicians. Our analysis of provider choice considers office-based, general-family practitioners and office-based specialists as alternatives. The result consistently emerges that families whose financial resources presumably allow them to purchase either tend to select office-based specialists.

In fact, the characteristics of patients of office-based general-family practitioners often appear to be more similar to those of patients of hospital-based providers. Judging from its actions, it is by no means certain that the American public is as convinced as are many policy-makers and experts in the health delivery field of the value of services rendered by general family physicians. We cannot rule out the possibility with current evidence that the public now views its choice as that between a technologically out-of-date general physician and the more recent vintage specialist. If so, public acceptance of the new breed of family physician may be higher.

A relationship between physician availability in a locality and provider choice has been clearly shown in this chapter. When physicians are scarce in relation to population, patient dependence on hospital-based sources of ambulatory care, including emergency room, rises substantially. Most experts in the health care field regard the use of the hospital for routine ambulatory care as undesirable. Thus, our finding with regard to physician availability implies that government efforts to improve the spatial distribution of physicians have beneficial impacts on access.

Notes

1. See, for example, Alberta W. Parker, "The Dimensions of Primary Care: Blueprints for Change," in Spyros Andreopoulos, *Primary Care,* New York: John Wiley and Sons, 1974, pp. 105–30.

2. P.R. Torrens and D.G. Yednab, "Variations Among Emergency Rooms: A Comparison of Four Hospitals in New York City," *Medical Care* 8 (January–February 1970):60–75; A. Jacobs, et al., "Emergency Department Utilization in an Urban Community," *Journal of the American Medical Association* 216 (April 12, 1971):307–312.

3. U.S. Department of Health, Education, and Welfare, National Center for Health Statistics, *Physician Visits and Interval Since the Last Visit, United States, 1969,* (Vital and Health Statistics) data from the *National Health Survey* 10 (75), Washington: U.S. Government Printing Office, 1972; Lu Ann Aday and Ronald Andersen, *Access to Medical Care,* Ann Arbor, Michigan: Health Administration Press, 1975.

4. Frank Sloan and Bruce Steinwald, "Variations in Appointment Delays for Physician Services: Theory and Empirical Evidence," mimeographed.

5. Victor Fuchs, *Who Shall Live?,* New York: Basic Books, Inc., 1974.

6. Cross-tabulations, based on MAS data, are presented in: The Robert Wood Johnson Foundation, *Special Report on Access—America's Health Care System: A Comprehensive Portrait,* Princeton, New Jersey, 1978.

7. A. James Lee, *Employment, Unemployment, and Health Insurance,* Cambridge, Massachusetts: Abt Books, 1979.

8. For example, a patient may be quite willing to incur the $5.00 additional charge of a physician with a low waiting time if an insurer is willing to pay $4.00 of the additional expense. See a study by Sloan and Lorant for a more complete discussion of this point: Frank Sloan and John Lorant, "The Role of Waiting Time: Evidence from Physicians' Practices," *Journal of Business* 50 (October 1977):486–507.

9. John K. Iglehart, "Jobless Medical Aid Debate Focuses on Financing Methods," *National Journal* (March 29, 1975):457–463.

10. Robert M. Gibson and Marjorie S. Mueller, "National Health Expenditures, Fiscal Year 1976," *Social Security Bulletin* 40 (April 1977):3–22.

11. Frank Sloan, Jerry Cromwell, and Janet Mitchell, *Private Physicians and Public Programs,* Lexington, Massachusetts: DC Heath-Lexington Books, 1978.

12. *Ibid.*

13. Frank Sloan, "The Demand for Physicians' Services in Alternative Practice Settings: A Multiple Logit Analysis," *Quarterly Review of Economics and Business* 18 (Spring 1978):41–61.

14. Sloan and Lorant, "The Role of Waiting Time."

15. Frank Sloan and John Lorant, "The Allocation of Physicians' Services: Evidence on Length of Visit," *Quarterly Review of Economics and Business* 16 (Autumn 1976):85–103.

16. Michael Grossman, *The Demand for Health: A Theoretical and Empirical Investigation,* New York: Columbia University Press, 1972.

17. For many purposes, the failure to consider stochastic changes in health status is not very important. As discussed below, our empirical measures of health differ from Grossman's. See Grossman, *The Demand for Health* and Michael Grossman and Lee Benham, "Health, Hours, and Wages," in Mark Perlman (ed.), *The Economics of Health and Medical Care,* London: MacMillan Press, 1974, pp. 679-694. Both studies used a measure of self-evaluated health status: health—excellent, good, fair, or poor. But it is not really clear what such a measure means. For example, as noted in chapter 1, a malingerer might report ill health as an excuse for not working or for poor performance on the job. If so, the measure's use as an explanatory variable in equations describing labor force activity and wages (as in Grossman and Benham) is questionable. The measures of restricted-activity days and bed-disability days is subject to a similar limitation since health may be given as an excuse for staying away from work. In this and the following chapter, our health status measures are based on specific symptoms reported by respondents.

18. Gary S. Becker, "A Theory of the Allocation of Time," *The Economic Journal* 75 (September 1965):493-517.

19. For more details of the MAS, see Robert Wood Johnson Foundation, *Special Report on Access*; Lu Ann Aday, Ronald Andersen, Gretchen Fleming, *A National Survey of Access to Medical Care* (forthcoming).

20. See an article by Porter for the circumstances under which weighted regression is desirable: Richard D. Porter, "On the Use of Survey Sample Weights in the Linear Model," *Annuals of Economic and Social Measurement* 2 (April 1973):141-58. Under certain plausible assumptions, weighted regression is not necessary.

21. A question on the dollar amount paid out of pocket for a visit was asked, but we decided not to use this information. Net price information was requested without reference to the procedures performed during the visit. Patients paying identical fees for specified procedures and having exactly the same insurance coverage could have very different net prices, depending on which services the physician rendered.

22. Reduced-fee service and bad debts were unimportant in the fee-for-service sector by the mid-1970s. See Sloan, Cromwell, and Mitchell, *Private Physicians.*

23. Job search time of the unemployed is low on average. See Arthur M. Okun, "Inflation: Its Mechanics and Welfare Costs," *Brookings Papers on Economic Activity* 2 (1975):351–401.

24. After careful examination, it appears that the problem lies not with our particular labor supply functions; labor supply functions reported in other studies, we have learned ex post, also generate implausible shadow wages. To our knowledge, however, ours is the first study to provide documentation.

25. For a "layman's" guide to discriminant analysis, see Norman H. Nie, et al., *SPSS: Statistical Package for the Social Sciences,* New York: McGraw-Hill, 1975.

26. They are slightly higher in the retiree regressions, which are based on smaller samples.

27. This is how the predicted probabilities are generated. Suppose there are n choices and x_i is a vector of individual characteristics and/or community characteristics pertaining to an individual, then the probability that the ith alternative is selected by a person with individual and/or community characteristics is expressed in logit analysis as:

$$P_i = e^{\alpha'_i x} \left/ \sum_{m=1}^{n} e^{\alpha'_m x} \right.$$

Classification functions from discriminant analysis often provide the starting values of the αs for logit analysis. As noted in the text, in our experience, classification function estimates tend to be quite close to final logit estimates. We use the above equation and our estimated classification functions to generate the predicted probabilities presented below.

28. The Part B proportions should be in the 0.9s rather than the 0.7s and 0.8s. We are unable to explain why in MAS some respondents failed to acknowledge their Part B coverage. Perhaps some respondents who had not received Part B benefits were not aware that they had such coverage.

29. Sloan, "Demand for Physicians' Services."

30. Sloan, Cromwell and Mitchell, *Private Physicians.*

6

Variations in Waiting Time, Length of Visit and Appointment Delays for Ambulatory Care

Our emphasis in this chapter is on the policy issues addressed at the beginning of chapter 5. As before, we are primarily interested in gauging the impacts of job loss, and the associated income and private insurance loss, on access to physicians' services. Our secondary objectives include assessing the access differences attributable to Medicaid coverage, race-ethnicity, and physician availability. As in chapters 4 and 5, our analysis is exclusively on the patient or the demand side of the market for ambulatory care. Even more specifically, we are concerned with those aspects of the access to such care as can be characterized by variations in length of visit, waiting time, and appointment delays for ambulatory care.

Among the process dimensions of access, lengths of visit, patient waits in physicians' office and clinics, and appointment delays have received as much attention by researchers as any other. Pertinent findings from past studies on these access indicators were reviewed in chapter 2. Recent accounts of trends in waiting time, length of visit, and appointment delays during the early to mid-1970s merit brief mention here.

According to Eisenberg, who estimated waiting time in private physicians' offices on the basis of annual surveys conducted by the American Medical Association, mean waiting time was 22.3 and 22.4 minutes in 1971 and 1973, respectively; in 1974 and 1975, it fell to 20.3 and 20.6 minutes, respectively. Eisenberg also presented estimates of mean appointment delays, based on the same data source; the mean delay rose from 5.1 days in 1971 to 8.7 days in 1973; then it declined to 7.3 days in 1974 and rose slightly in 1975.[1] Calculations based on data from annual AMA surveys presented by Bobula suggest that the national mean length rose slightly from 1973 to 1974-1975, although the trend in length of visit has been downward for the 1967-1975 period as a whole.[2] Thus, on balance, these data suggest that access, measured in terms of these three process indicators, improved slightly during 1974-1975. The period was characterized by slightly longer visits, less patient waiting time, and shorter appointment delays.

Do adverse economic conditions impact favorably on the process dimensions of access? Perhaps, but one must reflect on the other factors that might have influenced these results before one draws specific conclusions. Thus, for example, one should note that physicians' fees were controlled from late 1971 to early 1974 under the Economic Stabilization Program (ESP). Clearly, with prices controlled, physicians may have been forced to use nonprice rationing

131

methods during the ESP period. Later, when price was unconstrained by government controls, they may have relied more heavily on the price mechanism as a means for restraining demand. Thus, it is possible that the longer visits, shorter waiting time, and shorter appointment delays that obtained in 1974–1975 were but a manifestation of a shift in the relative importance of price and nonprice rationing.

The data source of our assessment of variations in waiting time, length of visit, and appointment delays is again the Medical Access Study (MAS). The theoretical concepts, definitions of explanatory variables, and methods for stratifying the MAS sample that apply in the present context have been discussed at length in chapter 5 and are further described in the appendix.

The MAS included questions on a number of process measures, including the three selected for analysis in this chapter. As in our analysis of patient choice of physician provider, the dependent variables are based on answers to questions about the respondent's "most recent visit." As noted in chapter 5, there are definite advantages to visit-specific access measures, as opposed to information based on the respondent's "usual source."

Although the case for using visit-specific information is strong on balance, there is also an important drawback. Random occurrences are likely to be far more prevalent in visit-specific responses. The patient may have had an unusually long wait because the physician was called out on an emergency; the last visit may have been very short because only a routine check on medication was involved; an appointment delay may have been unusually long because the physician took his annual summer vacation. Random elements in the dependent variables per se do not cause biased estimates; but the standard errors of estimated parameters may be larger, and the R^2s tend to be lower.

Since the pertinent theoretical framework, empirical specification of variables, and the samples have already been discussed in previous chapters, we can proceed immediately to our empirical results. Then we will relate our findings to previous work on these three variables and discuss policy implications.

Empirical Results

As we did in chapter 5, we have organized the tables of results around four samples: retirees, female heads of households; married men, and married women. Each table contains means, standard deviations, and regression results for each of the three dependent variables. Unlike chapter 5, in this section we shall discuss each of the three dependent variables in sequence. In each subsection, we will draw on results from each of the four tables.

Waiting Time

The waiting time regressions for the four samples are presented in tables 6–1 through 6–4. The dependent variable is measured in minutes.

The empirical results for retirees are contained in table 6-1. None of the coefficients in the waiting time regression (WAIT) are statistically significant at conventional levels in the retiree regression. However, two results are at least suggestive. First, with a t-ratio of 1.7, permanent nonearned income (NEYP) is nearly significant at the 5 percent level; the associated elasticity of -0.53 evaluated at the variable means implies a sizeable reduction in time spent waiting for physicians as permanent nonearned income rises. Second, the MCAID parameter estimate is positive and larger than its standard error. The parameter implies that Medicaid recipients wait twenty-six minutes longer than nonMedicaid recipients

Table 6-1
Waiting Time, Length of Visit, and Appointment Delay Regressions: Retirees

Variable	Means and Standard Deviations from			Regressions		
	WAIT Regression	LOV Regression	APPT Regression	WAIT	LOV	APPT
WAIT	44.20 (58.93)	– (–)	– (–)	– (–)	– (–)	– (–)
LOV	– (–)	20.79 (12.32)	– (–)	– (–)	– (–)	– (–)
APPT	– (–)	– (–)	2.14 (4.29)	– (–)	– (–)	– (–)
MDPC	11.51 (5.68)	11.66 (5.71)	10.81 (5.89)	−0.41 (9.60)	−0.49* (0.20)	0.02 (0.09)
MCAID	0.09 (0.29)	– (–)	– (–)	26.21 (19.44)	– (–)	– (–)
PARTB	0.78 (0.42)	0.78 (0.42)	0.74 (0.44)	−1.82 (13.44)	1.25 (2.72)	1.73* (1.33)
BLACK	0.12 (0.33)	0.11 (0.31)	0.13 (0.33)	2.36 (16.69)	7.22* (3.66)	0.34 (1.65)
NEYP	6886. (2719.)	6836. (2729.)	6491. (2555.)	−0.0034 (0.0020)	0.0005 (0.0004)	−0.0000 (0.0002)
RESID	−14.59 (3577.)	34.48 (3582.)	−149.8 (3309.)	−0.0009 (0.0015)	−0.0001 (0.0003)	−0.0001 (0.0002)
ASEV1	– (–)	0.11 (0.31)	0.15 (0.36)	– (–)	1.56 (4.61)	0.40 (2.49)
ASEV2	– (–)	0.07 (0.26)	0.10 (0.36)	– (–)	10.43* (5.14)	4.02 (2.63)
CSEV1	– (–)	0.52 (0.50)	0.54 (0.50)	– (–)	6.35 (3.52)	0.85 (2.15)
CHKUP	– (–)	0.18 (0.38)	0.14 (0.35)	– (–)	8.88* (4.21)	0.24 (2.60)
CONSTANT	– (–)	– (–)	– (–)	71.25 (–)	3.96 (–)	−0.25 (–)
				$R^2 = 0.06$ $F(6,116) = 1.2$	$R^2 = 0.14$ $F(9,113) = 2.1*$	$R^2 = 0.10$ $F(9,62) = 0.73$

*Significant at the 5 percent level

on the average; however, it must be noted that there are only eleven Medicaid recipients in the sample and therefore the results should be viewed as very tentative.

Two waiting time regressions based on the female head sample are presented in table 6-2; the only difference between the two is that the second includes HEM. The shadow wage for employed persons is the hourly market wage HDY; for the nonemployed, the shadow wage is HDY + α_1HDY. HEM represents α_1HDY. With a t-ratio of 1.88, HEM's coefficient is nearly significant at the 5 percent level. If the effects of both HDY and HEM are considered together, coefficients from the second regression imply that a female head, who during "normal" (nonrecessionary) times can earn $2.30 per hour (the federal minimum wage during 1975-1976), will wait for the doctor 6.9 minutes longer when she is not employed.

The coefficient RESID is negative and exceeds its standard error in the first equation and is significant at the 5 percent level in the second. RESID includes income from transfer payments, but is not limited to income from such sources. If the choice of physician is more responsive to permanent than to transitory income, one would expect the coefficients of permanent nonearned income (NEYP) to have a greater impact on waiting than that of RESID (since RESID incorporates transitory income). The opposite pattern, however, is observed in table 6-2. The RESID coefficients imply that an increase in transitory income, brought about for example by a rise in real public assistance payments, would lead to a reduction in female head waiting time. By contrast, the effect of NEYP on waiting time is essentially zero. The RESID coefficient implies that a $5,000 increase in transitory-residual income would reduce waiting time 6.5 minutes.

The physician-population ratio (MDPC) parameter estimates are negative in both waiting time regressions and nearly significant (with t-ratios of 1.86 and 1.88 respectively). Elasticities based on these coefficients are both −0.31; alternatively, if the patient care physician-population ratio were to rise from 2.5 per 10,000 population to the sample mean of 13.5 per 10,000, waiting time would fall by 3.4 minutes. The MDPC coefficients in table 6-2 are about three times as large in absolute value as those reported by Sloan and Lorant in their empirical analysis of waiting time based on a 1973 sample of physicians.[3]

Both private insurance variables, FCOV and PCOV, have anticipated negative coefficients in table 6-2, but only those for PCOV are sufficiently precise to merit any degree of confidence. As noted in chapter 5, we surmise from patterns (not reported in this study) that a high proportion of Medical Access Study respondents with full coverage were enrolled in independent plans (such as those operated by unions). The PCOV coefficients imply that female heads with partial coverage spend substantially less time waiting for physicians—twelve and nine minutes, respectively, according to the two regressions. The MCAID parameter estimates indicate no differences between female heads with Medicaid coverage and other female heads.

The BLACK coefficients suggest that black female heads spend considerably more time waiting than their white counterparts. Though positive, the

SURNAME coefficients are much smaller and far less precise. As noted in the appendix, the market wage (HDY) has been predicted from a wage-generating equation with race-ethnicity, inter alia, as an explanatory variable; so the results for blacks cannot be ascribed to black-white differences in the opportunity costs of time. A lack of physicians in the areas where black female heads work and live and/or discrimination are possible alternative explanations.

The results for married persons in table 6–3 confirm some of the preceding findings, but they also reflect some contradictions. As in the female head regressions, the MDPC parameter estimate in the case of married men is negative and is about two-thirds as large as the estimates for female heads. The BLACK coefficient is significant at the one percent level and the coefficient implies that black married men wait about twenty-eight minutes longer on the average than do their white counterparts. The NEYP and RESID parameter estimates are again negative; but as with female heads, the RESID estimate is the larger in absolute value. The major differences relate to PCOV and HDY; both were nearly significant in the female head regressions and explain essentially none of the variation in waiting time of married males.

Waiting time regressions for married women with and without the HEM and SEM variables are included in table 6–4. Neither HEM nor SEM are significant, but each coefficient exceeds its respective standard error and is positive. The positive SEM coefficient suggests that nonemployed women wait longer; likewise, wives of nonemployed husbands tend to wait longer. As noted in our discussion of patient choice of provider in chapter 5, nonemployment of the husband affected the wife's provider choice; however, nonemployment of the wife did not affect the husband's choice; nor did the husband's own employment status play a role in his own provider choice. The results presented in table 6–4 are certainly consistent with these earlier findings. The HEM and SEM coefficients would merit more confidence if HDY and SPY performed well in the WAIT regressions for married women. But, although the simple correlations are negative, the negative relationship largely disappears in the regression when all explanatory variables are included.

The MDPC parameter estimates are negative and significant at the 5 percent level. In terms of magnitude, they lie between those for married men and those for female heads. As in the married males case, private insurance demonstrates no effect on patient waits. Both BLACK and SURNAME coefficients are significant; the BLACK coefficients are approximately the same as those for female heads and about half as large as those for married men. The SURNAME variable only has a significant impact in the married women waiting time regressions. As in other regressions, RESID has a negative impact on patient waits.

Length of Visit

On the whole, both the length of visit and the appointment delay regressions perform less satisfactorily than the waiting time regressions. In order to avoid

Table 6-2
Waiting Time, Length of Visit, and Appointment Delay Regressions: Female Heads

	Means and Standard Deviations from:			Regressions					
Variable	WAIT Regressions	LOV Regressions	APPT Regressions	WAIT (1)	WAIT (2)	LOV (1)	LOV (2)	APPT (1)	APPT (2)
WAIT	39.74 (45.91)	— (—)	— (—)	— (—)	— (—)	— (—)	— (—)	— (—)	— (—)
LOV	— (—)	21.26 (14.77)	— (—)	— (—)	— (—)	— (—)	— (—)	— (—)	— (—)
APPT	— (—)	— (—)	5.11 (9.94)	— (—)	— (—)	— (—)	— (—)	— (—)	— (—)
MDPC	13.45 (5.42)	13.45 (5.43)	13.09 (5.33)	-0.91 (0.49)	-0.92 (0.48)	0.05 (0.16)	0.05 (0.16)	0.02 (0.11)	0.03 (0.11)
MCAID	0.19 (0.39)	0.19 (0.39)	0.19 (0.40)	0.51 (7.73)	-5.04 (8.24)	1.70 (2.49)	3.11 (2.66)	0.20 (1.80)	1.28 (1.92)
FCOV	0.06 (0.24)	0.06 (0.24)	0.06 (0.24)	-3.44 (11.20)	-1.41 (11.20)	2.75 (3.53)	2.24 (3.54)	3.66 (2.66)	3.27 (2.66)
PCOV	0.24 (0.43)	0.24 (0.43)	0.23 (0.42)	-11.76 (6.32)	-9.18 (6.44)	2.22 (2.01)	1.57 (2.05)	0.69 (1.49)	0.19 (1.52)
BLACK	0.24 (0.43)	0.24 (0.43)	— (—)	13.45† (6.69)	13.22† (6.67)	4.91† (2.12)	4.99† (2.12)	-5.70* (1.59)	-5.84* (1.58)
SURNAME	0.10 (0.31)	0.10 (0.30)	0.11 (0.32)	3.06 (9.29)	2.40 (9.26)	-1.62 (2.98)	-1.46 (2.97)	-4.75† (2.07)	-4.68† (2.06)
FSIZ	2.27 (1.65)	2.29 (1.65)	2.33 (1.67)	0.93 (1.91)	1.32 (1.91)	-1.12 (0.61)	-1.23† (0.61)	-0.01 (0.43)	-0.04 (0.43)
NEYP	1736. (1937.)	1750. (1939.)	1698. (1775.)	0.0005 (0.0014)	-0.0003 (0.0015)	-0.0003 (0.0005)	-0.00004 (0.0005)	0.0006 (0.0004)	0.0007 (0.0004)
RESID	-88.04 (4677.)	-88.34 (4674.)	-250.2 (4634.)	-0.0008 (0.0006)	-0.0013† (0.0006)	0.0004† (0.0002)	0.0005† (0.0002)	-0.0008 (0.00014)	0.0000 (0.0002)

	(1)	(2)	(3)	(4)	(5)	(6)	(7)	(8)	(9)
HDY	4.64 (1.61)	4.66 (1.60)	4.59 (1.66)	-2.44 (1.81)	-3.01 (1.83)	0.78 (0.58)	0.92 (0.58)	-0.65 (0.41)	-0.58 (0.41)
HEM	1.10 (1.99)	1.11 (2.00)	0.92 (1.77)	— (—)	3.01 (1.60)	— (—)	-0.76 (0.51)	— (—)	-0.67 (0.41)
ASEV1	— (—)	0.14 (0.35)	0.18 (0.39)	— (—)	— (—)	-4.35 (3.52)	-4.14 (3.52)	-2.27 (2.57)	-1.91 (2.56)
ASEV2	— (—)	0.18 (0.39)	0.17 (0.38)	— (—)	— (—)	-2.88 (3.35)	-2.61 (3.35)	-1.48 (2.54)	-1.33 (2.53)
CSEV1	— (—)	0.37 (0.48)	0.32 (0.47)	— (—)	— (—)	1.52 (3.07)	1.86 (3.07)	-1.71 (2.36)	-1.39 (2.36)
CHKUP	— (—)	0.22 (0.41)	0.24 (0.43)	— (—)	— (—)	5.56 (3.26)	5.77 (3.25)	8.61* (2.40)	8.77* (2.40)
CONSTANT	— (—)	— (—)	— (—)	59.74 (—)	60.04 (—)	17.36 (—)	17.04 (—)	7.22 (—)	7.16 (—)
				$R^2 = 0.07$ $F_{(10,304)} = 2.3*$	$R^2 = 0.08$ $F_{(11,303)} = 2.4*$	$R^2 = 0.12$ $F_{(14,298)} = 3.0*$	$R^2 = 0.13$ $F_{(15,297)} = 3.0*$	$R^2 = 0.27$ $F_{(14,207)} = 5.6*$	$R^2 = 0.28$ $F_{(15,206)} = 5.5*$

*Significant at 1 percent level; †significant at 5 percent level.

Table 6-3
Waiting Time, Length of Visit, and Appointment Delay Regressions: Married Males

Variable	*Means and Standard Deviations*			WAIT	LOV	APPT
	WAIT Regression	*LOV Regression*	*APPT Regression*			
WAIT	34.46	–	–	–	–	–
	(48.62)	(–)	(–)	(–)	(–)	(–)
LOV	–	20.96	–	–	–	–
	(–)	(19.60)	(–)	(–)	(–)	(–)
APPT	–	–	4.23	–	–	–
	(–)	(–)	(–)	(–)	(–)	(–)
MDPC	12.12	12.07	12.05	−0.61	0.16	0.10
	(5.11)	(5.10)	(5.18)	(0.42)	(0.16)	(0.10)
FCOV	0.07	0.07	0.07	2.55	0.39	5.38
	(0.26)	(0.26)	(0.25)	(8.40)	(3.30)	(2.13)
PCOV	0.44	0.44	0.43	−0.14	1.05	1.40
	(0.50)	(0.50)	(0.50)	(4.41)	(1.72)	(1.08)
VACOV	0.07	0.07	0.06	−1.35	3.22	−2.41
	(0.25)	(0.25)	(0.23)	(8.50)	(3.27)	(2.26)
BLACK	0.08	0.08	0.07	28.38*	2.70	−3.12
	(0.28)	(0.27)	(0.25)	(7.94)	(3.14)	(2.09)
SURNAME	0.08	0.08	0.09	6.71	2.49	−1.95
	(0.27)	(0.27)	(0.28)	(8.22)	(3.18)	(1.92)
FSIZ	3.69	3.67	3.71	−2.41	0.49	0.17
	(1.52)	(1.48)	(1.47)	(1.46)	(0.59)	(0.37)
NEYP	996.	991.	894.	−0.0001	0.0002	0.0002
	(2557.)	(2446.)	(2368.)	(0.0009)	(0.0003)	(0.0002)
RESID	−235.	−332.	−343.	−0.0005	−0.0002	0.00005
	(6093.)	(6076.)	(5963.)	(0.0004)	(0.0001)	(0.00009)
HDY	7.05	7.05	7.08	0.48	0.38	−0.05
	(2.13)	(2.15)	(2.17)	(1.23)	(0.48)	(0.30)
SPY	4.54	4.52	4.53	3.70†	0.83	0.37
	(1.67)	(1.67)	(1.67)	(1.45)	(0.56)	(0.35)
ASEV1	–	0.26	0.30	–	5.81	3.06
	(–)	(0.44)	(0.46)	(–)	(5.61)	(3.06)
ASEV2	–	0.22	0.19	–	3.52	−0.98
	(–)	(0.41)	(0.39)	(–)	(5.63)	(3.14)
CSEV1	–	0.32	0.29	–	7.15	0.68
	(–)	(0.47)	(0.45)	(–)	(5.55)	(3.06)
CHKUP	–	0.19	0.19	–	23.13*	9.24*
	(–)	(0.39)	(0.40)	(–)	(5.67)	(3.11)
CONSTANT	–	–	–	61.14	7.92	−0.84
	(–)	(–)	(–)	(–)	(–)	(–)
				$R^2=0.05$	$R^2=0.14$	$R^2=0.18$
				$F(11,523)=$	$F(15,504)=$	$F(15,402)=$
				2.4*	5.6*	5.7*

*Significant at 1 percent level; † significant at 5 percent level.

needless repetition of negative findings, we shall emphasize the more useful results. If we fail to mention a particular variable, the implication is that no meaningful relationship has been obtained.

The effects of wage-income variables on length of visit are most easily interpreted in the case of retirees and female heads. As retiree permanent income rises, length of visit (LOV) tends to rise. In contrast to the waiting time case, both earned and nonearned income only generate "pure" income effects on the length-of-visit dependent variable; price of time effects, potentially important in an analysis of waiting time, can be considered on a priori grounds to be inconsequential in this context. Although a longer visit takes more time of both the physician and the patient, it is doubtful that the patient considers time spent with the physician and his staff as wasteful.

Household head wage (HDY) coefficients are positive and exceed their standard errors in both female head regressions presented in table 6-2. Using the HDY coefficient from the second regression, the LOV-HDY elasticity (evaluated at the sample means) is 0.20. The coefficients of the RESID and NEYP variables are negative and positive, respectively—a positive sign was anticipated in both cases. If the HDY variable is converted from an hourly to a full-time annual salary, one can show that the HDY and RESID coefficients imply about the same magnitude of length-of-visit response to changes in female head income. The coefficient on HEM of −0.76 largely offsets the coefficient of 0.92 on HDY for nonemployed female heads. Again, assuming a $2.30 wage for female heads, the length of visit for nonemployed female heads is slightly under two minutes less than that of their employed counterparts.

The main noteworthy result on wage-income included in the married person tables is the significantly negative coefficient on SEM for married women. This is the only instance in the current context in which nonemployed married women appear to be at a disadvantage.

The family size (FSIZ) parameter estimates are negative in two out of the three sets of regressions in which they appear. When household income is held constant, larger families are poorer on a per capita basis. The largest FSIZ coefficient (see LOV(1) in table 6-4) has an associated elasticity of −0.13.

The physician availability (MDPC) coefficients are consistently positive, implying that physicians spend more time per visit with patients in communities with comparatively high physician-population ratios. The t-ratios corresponding to the MDPC coefficients exceed one in three of the four samples and indicate statistical significance at conventional levels in one of these. The largest parameter estimate is found in the case of retirees; the elasticity associated with it is 0.56.

The regressions suggest that blacks have longer visits on average, but the variable BLACK is only significant in the retiree and female head equations. Although this pattern may be taken to imply that blacks have better access than whites, measured in terms of length of visit, we cannot rule out the possi-

Table 6-4
Waiting Time, Length of Visit, and Appointment Delay Regressions: Married Females

Variable	Means and standard deviations from				Regressions					
	WAIT Regression	LOV Regression	APPT(1) Regression	APPT(2) Regression	WAIT(1)	WAIT(2)	LOV(1)	LOV(2)	APPT(1)	APPT(2)
WAIT	34.32 (39.77)	— (—)	— (—)	— (—)	— (—)	— (—)	— (—)	— (—)	— (—)	— (—)
LOV	— (—)	20.54 (15.09)	— (—)	— (—)	— (—)	— (—)	— (—)	— (—)	— (—)	— (—)
APPT	— (—)	— (—)	6.96 (17.90)	8.68 (19.63)	— (—)	— (—)	— (—)	— (—)	— (—)	— (—)
MDPC	12.24 (5.50)	12.24 (5.49)	12.22 (5.51)	12.70 (5.29)	-0.75† (0.31)	-0.72† (0.31)	0.26† (0.12)	0.26† (0.12)	-0.12 (0.16)	-0.24 (0.21)
FCOV	0.06 (0.23)	0.06 (0.23)	0.05 (0.21)	0.05 (0.22)	3.53 (7.13)	3.69 (7.13)	1.65 (2.71)	1.29 (2.71)	4.82 (4.01)	5.17 (4.80)
PCOV	0.41 (0.49)	0.41 (0.49)	0.42 (0.49)	0.43 (0.50)	0.27 (3.33)	0.78 (3.35)	0.25 (1.27)	0.39 (1.28)	0.55 (1.72)	0.39 (2.12)
BLACK	0.10 (0.31)	0.10 (0.30)	0.08 (0.27)	0.06 (0.24)	13.07† (5.64)	13.31† (5.66)	0.46 (2.17)	0.002 (2.17)	-3.16 (3.21)	-1.91 (4.42)
SURNAME	0.10 (0.31)	0.10 (0.30)	0.12 (0.32)	0.08 (0.28)	13.98† (5.76)	13.85† (5.75)	-2.32 (2.22)	-2.44 (2.21)	-5.04 (2.84)	-4.75 (3.89)
FSIZ	3.96 (1.55)	3.97 (1.54)	4.05 (1.54)	4.02 (1.51)	1.58 (1.08)	1.82 (1.09)	-0.72 (0.41)	-0.69 (0.41)	0.50 (0.55)	0.61 (0.70)
NEYP	701. (2198.)	700. (2199.)	665. (2176.)	742. (2134.)	0.0004 (0.0008)	0.0002 (0.0008)	-0.0005 (0.0003)	-0.0004 (0.0003)	0.0006 (0.0004)	0.0008 (0.0005)
RESID	-302. (5971.)	-307. (5967.)	-147. (5968.)	83. (6095.)	-0.0003 (0.0003)	-0.0005 (0.0003)	0.00001 (0.00010)	0.00010 (0.00011)	0.0002 (0.0001)	0.0002 (0.0002)
HDY	6.77 (2.23)	6.78 (2.24)	6.86 (2.36)	7.08 (2.34)	-0.80 (0.94)	-0.86 (0.94)	0.15 (0.36)	0.13 (0.36)	-0.49 (0.47)	-0.59 (0.57)

HEM	0.40 (1.59)	0.39 (1.58)	0.35 (1.50)	0.33 (1.47)	— (—)	1.67 (1.04)	0.17 (0.40)	— (—)	— (—)	— (—)
SPY	4.45 (1.67)	4.45 (1.67)	4.48 (1.69)	4.61 (1.61)	0.27 (1.12)	0.04 (1.16)	-0.14 (0.44)	-0.41 (0.43)	0.41 (0.58)	0.33 (0.73)
SEM	2.32 (2.46)	2.32 (2.46)	2.27 (2.47)	2.33 (2.51)	— (—)	0.87 (0.73)	-0.62 (0.28)	— (—)	— (—)	— (—)
ASEV1	— (—)	0.14 (0.35)	0.17 (0.38)	0.16 (0.36)	— (—)	— (—)	-3.38 (2.67)	-3.20 (2.26)	-8.81† (3.55)	-8.95† (4.32)
ASEV2	— (—)	0.16 (0.37)	0.17 (3.38)	0.17 (0.37)	— (—)	— (—)	0.41 (2.61)	0.44 (2.62)	-7.76† (3.54)	-7.95† (4.26)
CSEV1	— (—)	0.39 (0.49)	0.35 (0.48)	0.33 (0.47)	— (—)	— (—)	0.71 (2.35)	0.52 (2.35)	-3.57 (3.28)	-2.47 (3.94)
CHKUP	— (—)	0.23 (0.42)	0.23 (0.42)	0.27 (0.44)	— (—)	— (—)	3.85 (2.50)	3.85 (2.51)	4.77 (3.45)	5.26 (4.75)
CONSTANT	— (—)	— (—)	— (—)	— (—)	37.90 (—)	35.29 (—)	20.82 (—)	20.65 (—)	10.92 (—)	13.49 (—)
					$R^2 = 0.04$ $F(10,612) = 2.8*$	$R^2 = 0.05$ $F(12,610) = 2.6*$	$R^2 = 0.05$ $F(16,607) = 2.1*$	$R^2 = 0.04$ $F(14,609) = 2.0†$	$R^2 = 0.09$ $F(14,442) = 3.3*$	$R^2 = 0.09$ $F(14,351) = 2.5*$

*Significant at 1 percent level; †significant at 5 percent level.

bility that the MAS length-of-visit variables include some time that patients actually spend waiting for the physician. To the extent that this is so, the length-of-visit results would be consistent with our earlier findings that blacks wait longer. Moreover, this form of measurement error would also explain the poor results on wages and income in some of the length-of-visit regressions and is consonant with the fact that the MAS length-of-visit means are somewhat higher than estimates from the National Ambulatory Care Survey (NAMCS).

Tables 6-1 through 6-4 consistently report mean visit lengths of twenty-one minutes versus fourteen minutes for the 1973-1974 NAMCS.[4] The MAS asked the patient, "How much time did the doctor spend with you when you saw him?" The NAMCS obtains length-of-visit data from a "Patient Record" completed by the physician after the visit has taken place. The patient would probably be more likely to include time spent in an examining room waiting for the physician and/or his staff; unfortunately, we have no way of verifying this. Since we screened out visits lasting over two hours from our MAS sample prior to estimation and there is no reason to believe that such a screen was applied to the NAMCS, the difference between the NAMCS and the MAS is probably understated.

Judging from the *MCAID* coefficients in the female head regressions (the only *LOV* regressions in which this variable appears), Medicaid enrollees have longer visits. This result, however, is subject to the potential limitation just discussed in the context of black-white differences.

Appointment Delays

The MAS asked respondents, "Did you have an appointment (for the most recent visit) ahead of time or did you just walk in?" The respondent could answer "had appointment" or "walked in." For persons with an appointment, the MAS asked, "Did you set up this appointment at an earlier visit or call for an appointment at the time you needed to see the doctor?" If the patient called for an appointment, he was asked, "How long did you have to wait between the time you called for the appointment and the date you actually saw the doctor?"

We have defined two appointment delay dependent variables, both measured in days. Generally, the dependent variable reflects walk-ins, who are assumed to have an appointment delay of zero, and those who had scheduled visits; the one exception is the second appointment delay regression in table 6-4—in that one case, walk-ins have been excluded. In all cases, appointments scheduled at the previous visit have been excluded.

The mean appointment delay for retirees is slightly over two days. If walk-ins are excluded, a calculation not shown, the mean delay for retirees is slightly over three days. Given this very short delay, it is not surprising that the retiree appointment delay regression presented in table 6-1 offers no meaningful implications.

Two results from the female household regression in table 6-2 are noteworthy. First, blacks and Spanish-surnamed individuals experience shorter delays. This result persists when walk-ins are excluded (in regressions not shown). Second, there is no consistent pattern among the wage-income coefficients. While the negative coefficient on the wage (HDY) is negative, suggesting that short appointment delays are a normal good, the $NEYP$ and HEM parameter estimates offer the opposite implication.

The regressions for married persons presented in tables 6-3 and 6-4 more or less support the findings for female heads. The regressions imply that blacks and Spanish-surnamed among married individuals tend to experience shorter delays. Moreover, the coefficients of the wage and income variables also display no consistent pattern in these regressions.

As noted in chapter 2, Sloan and Steinwald hypothesized that a short appointment delay is a normal good, that is, it is more likely to be demanded by high income families.[5] They argued that poor persons see physicians for acute visits with greater frequency; by contrast, the visit mix of the more affluent reflects greater use of preventive services. Since the utility of immediate care is far greater for the former than for the latter visit type, it is not surprising that two-way tabulations, which do not control for diagnosis, often show appointment delays to be longer for the comparatively affluent. When they held diagnosis constant, Sloan and Steinwald found evidence in support of their hypothesis. The appointment delay regressions in tables 6-1 through 6-4 roughly hold diagnosis constant since reason-for-visit variables are included. We did not find a negative relationship between income and appointment delays in our analysis of MAS data, although we had anticipated that we might on the basis of Sloan-Steinwald's research.

Summary and Conclusions

In this chapter we have assessed three process dimensions of access: the amount of time that patients spent waiting for the physician; the amount of time that physicians spent with patients on a per visit basis; and the interval between the time that an appointment was made and the actual visit. According to the theory underlying our empirical analysis, persons with high opportunity costs of time eschew physicians who make them wait. Moreover, higher family "ability-to-pay" causes increased demand for "amenities," which include the reductions in waiting time, more contact with physicians, and ready access to physicians when the patient wants to see and/or talk with him. Ability-to-pay reflects both family income—adjusted for family size—and insurance coverage for ambulatory care.

As we noted at the outset of this chapter, national estimates of recent trends in all three process variables point in one direction. Access to physicians' services, as measured by these three variables, improved somewhat in 1974-1975 relative to 1973. In terms of waiting time, access appears to have been better in 1974-1975 than in 1971, but in terms of appointment delay and length of visit, access appears to have been better in the early than in the mid-1970s. The improvement in access in 1974-1975 may reflect the fact that price controls were eliminated in early 1974 and the trends may have little or nothing to do with the adverse economic conditions of 1974-1975. An examination of a few aggregate time series observations does not permit one to discriminate among alternative hypotheses regarding the causes of observed trends.

The Medical Access Study (MAS), a cross-sectional view of access covering a large national sample of households and individuals, permits an assessment of these three dimensions of access from the demand side of the physicians' services market. Without knowledge of the supply side, one cannot use demand side results to project aggregate trends in access. But one can assess changes on the demand side that are likely to lead to changes in aggregate behavior. Furthermore, our analysis has allowed us to examine access of particular groups, such as persons without jobs.

Evidence from past studies on all three process dimensions, briefly reviewed in chapter 2, is consistent with the theory that we have presented. Past findings clearly demonstrate that waiting time is longer in communities in which people on the average have low opportunity wages. Income and insurance have been found to be related to the demand for amenities in past work.

Clearly there is substantial variation in responses among the four dimensions of access considered in this and the preceding chapter and across the four demographic groups. In general, the results that concern patient choice of provider type and patient waiting time at the site of care are more informative than those that concern the length of visit and appointment delay.

There are several principal results of our waiting time analysis that relate to the policy issues addressed at the outset of chapter 5. There is *some* evidence that patients with high opportunity wages secure services from physicians who do not require lengthy waits. This pattern is particularly evident in our analysis of female heads of households and, to a much lesser extent, in results for married women. The regressions for married men do not reveal a meaningful relationship between wages and waiting. The female head results are sufficiently good in this regard to permit the inference that job loss leads to increased patient waits (for persons in this demographic category). Results for married persons simply do not support this conclusion. One might speculate that the relationship between waiting and wage-income is weaker in the higher part of the range of wage-income. Respondents in our married persons' samples tend to be far more affluent than are those in our female heads' sample.

We evaluated the effect of private health insurance in three out of the four samples, that is, all except retirees. Again, results consistent with our expectations have been obtained only in the case of female heads. Private insurance demonstrates a zero effect on waiting time of married persons. Therefore, we cannot conclude that loss of insurance coinciding with job loss affects waiting time as a general matter. But we can point to a specific instance in which private insurance seems to have had an effect. This finding contrasts with earlier work on waiting time by Sloan and Lorant.[6] The Sloan-Lorant study reported that private health insurance has an important negative impact on waiting time; they found waits were shorter in communities in which a high proportion of the population was insured for physicians' services.

A consequence of recession is increased dependence on the part of many citizens on public assistance in general and Medicaid in particular. For numerous reasons, physicians as a group have not been very receptive to Medicaid. Consequently, the Medicaid recipient may not fare as well in the health care system as his nonMedicaid counterpart. Certainly, it is reasonable to suppose that the Medicaid recipient is less likely to be offered amenities, as we use the term. We have attempted to gauge Medicaid effects on waiting when the sample size was sufficient to do so. We found that Medicaid patients have much longer waits in the retiree sample, but we found no difference in our sample of female heads.

We have assessed differences in waiting that relate to race and ethnicity. The coefficient for the variable BLACK is positive in all waiting time regressions and is almost always statistically significant at conventional levels. Precisely why blacks wait longer cannot be determined. However, one cannot attribute the relationship to lower wage-income of blacks. Ability-to-pay influences are held constant by other explanatory variables. The coefficients for the Spanish-surname variables are slightly less precise, but one can reasonably infer from our regressions that, holding other factors constant, Spanish-surnamed adults wait longer.

The regressions imply quite consistently that patients wait less in communities with high physician-population ratios. In view of the substantial amount of public funds devoted to improving the spatial distribution of physicians, this is a result worth emphasizing.

In view of the ambiguities of the length-of-visit and appointment delay results, it is inappropriate to list findings in a serial fashion. Therefore, we shall be very brief.

The regressions yield some evidence that the poor have shorter visits on the average. The physician-population ratio coefficients imply that visits are in fact longer where physicians are more numerous in relation to population. Essentially no link is found between private health insurance and visit length. As we noted in the last section, we suspect that an empirical analysis of length of visit would have been more successful if a more accurately measured dependent variable had been available. In future surveys, it would be desirable to design a more specific length-of-visit question.

Although the problem with the length-of-visit analysis appears to be primarily empirical, future work on appointment delays should begin with emphasis on the underlying concepts. We have assumed that a short delay is an amenity that consumers purchase as they become richer. That is, wealthier individuals find physicians who will see them, or at least speak with them, on reasonably short notice. Earlier research by Sloan and Steinwald supports this view,[7] but we found little supporting evidence in our analysis. Perhaps appointment delays must be viewed as being consumed jointly with waits in the physician's office. There may be a tradeoff between the two types of waiting and the more affluent may face this tradeoff on more favorable terms, but nevertheless may experience longer appointment delays.

It is difficult from the standpoint of public policy to state unequivocally what constitutes a "bad," or lengthy, appointment delay. Even so, the mean appointment delay of two days reported by retiree respondents to the Medical Access Study does not seem very high. The mean delays of four to seven days, reported for the other three groups, also would not appear to be especially alarming. However, while the appointment delay means are clearly not alarming, they may obscure lengthy delays for a few illnesses that would benefit from earlier treatment. Further research should seek to determine whether or not this is so.

Notes

1. Barry S. Eisenberg, "Non-Price Rationing: Evidence on Waiting Times and Price Controls," in Sharon R. Henderson (ed.), *Profile of Medical Practice,* Chicago: American Medical Association, 1977, pp. 65-72.

2. Joel D. Bobula, "Recent Trends in Physician Productivity," in Sharon R. Henderson (ed.), *Profile of Medical Practice,* Chicago: American Association, 1977, pp. 23-30.

3. Frank Sloan and John Lorant,"The Role of Waiting Time: Evidence from Physicians' Practices," *Journal of Business* 50 (October):486-507, 1977.

4. James E. DeLozier and Raymond O. Gagnon, *The National Ambulatory Medical Care Survey: 1973 Summary, United States 1973-April 1974,* Washington: Department of Health, Education, and Welfare, National Center for Health Statistics, 1976, DHEW Publication No. (HRA) 76-1772.

5. Frank Sloan and Bruce Steinwald, "Variations in Appointment Delays for Physician Services: Theory and Empirical Evidence, *Policy Sciences* (forthcoming).

6. Sloan and Lorant, "The Role of Waiting Time."

7. Sloan and Steinwald, "Variations in Appointment Delays."

7 Concluding Remarks

Since the mid-1960s there has been a substantial public effort directed towards the objective of improving the equity of access to medical care in the United States. In particular, Medicaid and Medicare have sought to eliminate financial barriers to the access to health care. Furthermore, there has been widespread support for medical education and for programs directed at improved organization and availability of medical manpower that attempt to redress geographical inequities. Additional effort has been focused on eliminating information barriers. Thus, for over a decade much of the health care policy in this country has been concerned with the equity of access to medical care. Although recent studies of the access to health care services emphasize that the current situation is far from ideal, these studies indicate that the trends in several access indicators, such as the number of physician visits and health-adjusted physician utilization rates, are encouraging.

In this study, we have attempted to identify and evaluate the impact of the adverse changes in aggregate economic conditions on the access to physicians. Have the secular trends in improved access been partially—or fully—reversed by the high rates of inflation and unemployment during this period? If so, have the low income and minority groups been predominately affected?

In order to answer these questions, we have reviewed the pertinent literature on patient access to ambulatory care, and undertaken various analyses of time-series and cross-sectional data. A multidimensional consideration of access to care has provided the conceptual framework for the empirical analysis. Each dimension captures a particular aspect of the delivery of ambulatory health care services. Indeed, the utilization of physicians' services, utilization relative to need, process measures, and indicators of patient satisfaction with care received, are all commonly accepted access measures, but they do not always offer the same implications. Therefore, this study considers all of these measures of access and subjects them to formal modeling based on unpublished data from the 1969-1975 Health Surveys conducted by the National Center for Health Statistics, and the Medical Access Study, conducted in 1975 by the Center for Health Administration Studies and the National Opinion Research Center, both affiliated with the University of Chicago.

In the context of the research undertaken in this study, the following indicators were subjected to analysis: physician visits; physician visits relative to health status measures; whether or not the patient has a usual source of physicians' services; whether or not the patient has encountered one or more problems obtaining medical care; unmet needs reported by patients; the patient's choice of physician provider; patient waits in the physician's office; length of time the physician spent with the patient during a recent visit; and the delay between the time the patient made an appointment and the actual visit.

Viewed in its entirety, the evidence shows a definite link between the performance of the economy on the one hand and patient access to physicians' services on the other. However, the effects of the former on the latter are not dramatic. Certainly we do not expect that future periods of inflation and recession will result in a total reversal of the gains in access realized during the preceding decade.

A first group of findings are evident from aggregate data. These results emerge rather quickly, without detailed cross-tabulations or multivariate analysis.

During the inflation-recession of the 1970s, unemployment constituted a greater threat to low income families than did inflation. Inasmuch as the value of transfer payments, such as Medicaid and other public assistance programs, was essentially preserved in real terms, persons on fixed incomes were insulated from the erosion of purchasing power that often results from inflation. Meaningful differences in cost-of-living increases among lower, intermediate, and higher budget families were not apparent from cost-of-living data. On the other hand, nonemployment income available through public programs only partly offsets income losses directly attributable to job loss. For this reason, persons who lost their jobs tended to be worse off, even though the purchasing power of transfer payments per se appears to have been preserved. Furthermore, during the 1974–1975 recession, there was a widespread loss of job-related health insurance which was greater for young, nonwhite, and female workers—groups which were heavily represented in the "disadvantaged" cohort.

Although the mean number of physician visits crept upward from 1969 through 1975, during the same period health-status adjusted utilization rates either remained the same or manifested a downward trend, depending on the health status measure used. Thus, although the mean number of physician visits increased, the number of sick days increased at least as fast.

Also during 1969–1975, there was a change in the choice of site of physician contact. The proportion of total visits occurring in hospital outpatient departments increased during this period. By contrast, there was a decrease in home visits as a percentage of total visits. On the basis of tabulations alone, it is difficult to attribute these changes to the performance of the economy. However, the regression analysis undertaken in this study establishes a relationship between patients' financial circumstances and their choice of site of ambulatory care. Many would view increased dependence on the hospital for ambulatory care as a negative development and one worthy of policymakers' attention.

There is evidence that patient waiting time in physicians' offices in 1974–1975 was about 10 percent below 1971–1973 levels. Mean appointment delays also fell in 1974–1975 from 1973 levels, but compared with 1971, the 1974–1975 mean is higher. The mean length of visit rose slightly from 1973, but considering the 1969–1975 period as a whole, a distinct trend toward shorter visits is suggested. Thus, on these criteria, recent trends in access are mixed.

Comparisons between the employed and unemployed show the latter to be far worse off in terms of several utilization, process, and satisfaction dimensions of access. For example, our data indicate that unemployed persons have 34 percent more visits per capita than their employed counterparts. However, dividing visits by our two measures of current disability, the unemployed appear to have much lower levels of access to physicians' services. Contrasts between employed and unemployed are also evident in our regression analysis, but they are not as large.

A comparison of the status of various dimensions of access between the first and fourth quarters of 1974 showed no meaningful changes in access over that year. By contrast, however, prices rose at double-digit rates throughout the year, and unemployment rates increased dramatically, especially in the fourth quarter. This result suggests that, although economic conditions prevailing in 1974 were far from ideal, they were not sufficiently bad to cause a rapid deterioration in patient access for the U.S. population as a whole.

Although highly aggregated data permitted analysis of the secular trends delineated above, they did not show sufficient cyclical variation to permit inferences relating to a more detailed perspective on the relationship between access to medical care and adverse economic conditions. Consequently, this study contains several multivariate models that serve as bases of additional analyses of several dimensions of access. Regression analyses resulted in findings regarding the utilization and need dimensions of access.

From regressions based on a time series, we estimate that real per capita income exerts a strongly positive impact on utilization. The estimates of income elasticities range from 0.4 to 1.3. These estimates tend to be higher than income elasticities obtained by others, but these differences can be reconciled. The other, lower estimates are based on a cross-sectional analysis; the estimates in this study are based on a time-series analysis. Only time-series data can isolate the tendency to defer some types of care during cyclical downturns. Our income elasticities reflect this factor, as well as the more long-run tendency, to consume more medical care as income rises.

Both inflation and unemployment have adverse impacts on health status, and thus are significant indirect determinants of utilization. This study confirms Brenner's findings that inflation and unemployment adversely influence health status.[1] Much more detailed empirical analysis of these relationships should be conducted, but at least as tentative conclusion, it is reasonably safe to say that an effect of adverse conditions in the economy is increased short-term disability.

Inflation has a negative direct effect on the number of physicians' visits. In view of the previously discussed findings that inflation also causes restricted activity and bed disability days to increase and thereby has a positive indirect effect on physician utilization, the indirect and direct effects work against each other. This study concludes that the negative direct effect and positive indirect effect essentially offset each other and result in a net effect of inflation equal to zero.

Unemployment exerts a weakly positive direct effect on the utilization of physicians' services. But we also find that the stress-related effects of unemployment lead to increased numbers of disability and restricted-activity days. The combined impact of both the direct and indirect effects of unemployment on utilization of physicians' services is positive, reflecting the propensity for the two effects to reinforce each other.

Cross-sectional data have provided the basis for the analysis of process and satisfaction dimensions of access. In general, we conclude that the type of ambulatory medical care that individuals receive partially reflects prevailing economic conditions. More specific findings emerge from the cross-sectional regression analysis of patient's usual source of care, problems obtaining medical care, and self-perceived unmet health care needs.

In terms of the presence of problems obtaining medical care and unmet needs, the long-term unemployed have worse access than their short-term unemployed counterparts—although the differences between the long- and short-term unemployed and between the unemployed and employed are small. Family income consistently demonstrates negative effects on these process and satisfaction measures. Clearly the poor are worse off. Combining job loss with family income loss results in larger loss in access than either one in isolation. Educational attainment shows at most a small impact on access.

In general, the results based on regression analysis of summary process and satisfaction measures of access imply that the adverse effects on access should be counted in any itemization of the costs of unemployment. Yet, because unemployment and income explain only a small portion of the variation in these dependent variables and the associated elasticities are small, there is no reason to believe that if the economy were to achieve full employment, all access problems would be solved. Our table, based on cross-tabulations, implies that unemployment is a more important factor in access differentials than do our regressions. When the two conflict, the regression results merit more attention.

Discriminant analysis of provider choice has led to further implications regarding process and satisfaction dimensions of access. In particular, this study considered patients' choices of site of care. Such choices have important implications for access. Continuity of care is less likely when the patient relies on hospital based sources of ambulatory care as opposed to office-based care. There is also evidence that patient waits are longer in hospital settings as are appointment delays for patients who make appointments. The analysis in this study assessed patient choice among two types of office-based and two types of hospital-based providers of ambulatory care services. Furthermore, this analysis has provided a useful perspective for considering the sources of the growth in the relative importance of hospital outpatient clinics and emergency rooms. Some of the important results from this analysis follow.

There is substantial variation in the behavioral relationships among the four samples analyzed: retirees, female heads of household; married men; and married women. Retirees are aged 65 and over; ages of all others range from 25 to 64. In general, the choices of retirees and female household heads are associated more closely with financial variables than are the choices of married persons. This result may be attributed to two factors. First, retiree and female heads tend to have lower incomes. The underlying relationships may be non-linear with "economic" variables playing a more dominant role in the lower ranges. Second, the variants in the basic model used in the retiree and female head analysis are comparatively simple, and hence more easily interpreted. From the vantage point of policy, the results emphasize the danger of generalizing from the "average" behavior of several heterogeneous groups.

The relationship between nonearned income and provider choice is far clearer for retirees and female heads of households probably because these groups are typically far more dependent on income from nonemployment sources. Based on this finding, this analysis establishes a link between transfer payment programs, such as Social Security and Aid to Families with Dependent Children, and the provider choice of dimension of access. Cuts in real Social Security and/or AFDC benefits would cause these groups to rely more on hospital as opposed to office-based medical care.

Nonemployed female household heads are more likely, holding other factors constant, to use hospital sources of ambulatory care. By contrast, non-employment of married men has no impact on their own provider choices, but their wives do tend to rely more heavily on hospital sources of ambulatory care.

Although the role of inflation-recession is principally emphasized in this brief review of major findings, another access determinant certainly merits mention. The provider choice results consistently show a direct relationship between physician availability and the kind of provider chosen by the patient. For example, if one type of physician is a rarity in a particular community, patients will substitute other physicians for the scarce variety. Moreover, when physicians are scarce in relation to population, patient dependence in hospital-based sources of ambulatory care, including emergency rooms, rises substantially. This finding implies that governmental efforts to improve the spatial distribution of physicians have substantial and beneficial impacts on access.

Sometimes, findings of no relationship when one was clearly expected is informative in its own right. It is widely held that many office-based physicians refuse to see Medicaid patients. We fail to find a systematic relationship between the Medicaid payment source and the patient's site of care. Perhaps, the results reflect the fact that our samples include few Medicaid patients; or perhaps, the Medicaid patients in our sample live in states with comparatively generous

Medicaid programs. We cannot say for sure, but the evidence should make one somewhat cautious about stating that the Medicaid patient has inadequate access to the office-based physician. Moreover, our results with regard to race-ethnicity and choice of site of care are inconclusive. Again, one cannot say from this study that blacks and Spanish-Americans are barred from office-based practices directly because of their racial or ethnic backgrounds. In both the Medicaid and race-ethnicity cases, it could be ability to pay that is mainly responsible for patients' choices.

We have also conducted multivariate analysis of time spent by patients waiting for the doctor, the length of visit, and delays between the date an appointment is made and the actual visit. Overall, the results pertaining to patient waiting time are much more informative than the findings from the length-of-visit and appointment delay analysis. The principal results of the waiting time analysis indicate that persons with lower opportunity wages (or equivalently, a lower cost of waiting) typically wait longer than persons with higher opportunity wages. This pattern is particularly evident in analyses of female heads of households. These results are sufficiently robust to permit the inference that job loss leads to increased patient waits for persons in this demographic cohort.

In addition, we hypothesized that insured persons tend to wait less than noninsured persons. This relationship is evident in analyses of female heads of households, but not for married men or women. At least for the female heads category, it is possible to infer that to the extent unemployment leads to the loss of health insurance, access is adversely affected.

On the whole, our waiting time regressions permit the conclusion the blacks and Spanish-surname individuals have longer waits in doctors' offices. Although this conclusion is stronger than the one involving race-ethnicity and choice of site, as before, our results on the Medicaid variable are conflicting. We are *not* able to say that, holding other variables such as family income constant, Medicaid patients wait longer.

An assessment of physician availability revealed that waiting is lower in communities with high physician-population ratios. This result reinforces our conclusion with regard to physician availability and patient choice of site of ambulatory care.

Scholars like to close their studies with pleas for more research. Granting that such pleas are often justified, it must also be said that studies are the scholar's stock in trade. Future research is clearly warranted on patient access to ambulatory care, especially empirical tests of relatively new theories of household decisionmaking as they relate to access. But this statement should not obscure the fact that a substantial amount of information has been assembled in this and several other studies.

At the time of this writing, the United States is in the midst of renewed inflation and the prospect of another "corrective" recession. On the basis of this study, we can say with considerable confidence that if inflation-recession is maintained within the bounds of the 1974-1975 experience, there will be little effect on access. As far as the U.S. population taken as a whole is concerned, the effect would be virtually nil; but there may well be access impacts on the groups most affected by adverse economic circumstances.

On the whole, the descriptive evidence presented in earlier chapters and briefly reviewed in this chapter, supports the findings of previous studies. Conceptual and multivariate analysis of access variables is much newer and more difficult, and hence our conclusions have frequently been more uncertain.

At this point, one important contribution of multivariate analysis is to make one more conservative about the effects of specific variables, certainly more so than one would be on the basis of the tabulations alone. Our emphasis through-out has been on an economic approach to access. Since economists have rarely dealt with many of these specific issues, this book has, hopefully, at least partly corrected an imbalance. There are many subtleties in household decisions pertaining to health care use. Ultimately, only with several disciplines working in concert will it be possible to fully understand the behavior evident in the surveys analyzed in this and other studies.

Notes

1. M. Harvey Brenner, *Estimating Social Costs of National Economic Policy: Implications for Mental and Physical Health and Criminal Aggression*, Washington: Joint Economic Committee of the U.S. Congress, October 26, 1976.

Appendix
Wage and Income
Variables for
Chapters 5 and 6

The Medical Access Study (MAS) analyzed in chapters 5 and 6 has many desirable features. A major deficiency, however, is its lack of detail on wages and income. In fact, the MAS only requested information on family income and asked if the respondent had *any* income from a list of sources furnished by the interviewer.

In this appendix, we show how the meager amount of "economic" information provided by the MAS was used to estimate the market *and* shadow wages for husband and wife and the permanent nonearned *and* transitory nonearned income of the family. The estimates of market wages and nonearned income are used in access regressions presented in chapters 5 and 6. We judged our shadow wage estimates to be too imprecise; hence, we used an approximation based on the market wage estimates in chapters 5 and 6. The good performance of the market wage and nonearned income variables in the labor supply regressions presented here gives us reason to believe that we have obtained reasonable estimates of these variables. Hence any anomalous findings with respect to ways and incomes in the two chapters are not easily blamed on inaccurate wage and income variables.

Methodology

Measured income (Y) may be subdivided into: (1) the household's permanent earned income (EY^*), (2) the household's permanent nonearned income (NEY^*), and (3) a residual (R) incorporating transitory income.

$$Y = EY^* + NEY^* + R \qquad (A.1)$$

Permanent earned income may be further classified into components attributable to adult male and female family members:

$$EY^* = EY_m^* + EY_f^* \qquad (A.2)$$

where m and f signify adult males and females, respectively.

The Medical Access Study (MAS) contains a measure of the family's *total combined income* (Y) for the year preceding the interview, and a checklist of income sources but no amounts by source.

The sources included in the checklist and the acronyms that we have assigned to each are:

Interest and dividends   = INTDIV

Rent   = RENT

Social Security retirement   = SSR

Social Security survivors   = SSI

Private pensions   = PP

Friends or relatives   = FR

Alimony or child support   = ACS

Armed forces allotment   = AFA

Unemployment compensation = UC

Workmen's Compensation   = WC

Public Aid   = PA

Veteran's Administration   = VA

Other   = OTH

If we treat each of the above sources, for the moment, as continuous income variables (rather than binaries), then:

$$NEY^* = \text{INTDIV} + \text{RENT} + \text{SSR} + \text{SSI} + \text{PP} + \text{ACS}$$
$$+ \text{AFA} + \text{VA} \tag{A.3}$$

According to equation A.3, all public assistance income is considered to be transitory.

Since the survey does not provide information on unearned income by source, we were forced to use dummy variable approximations; these dummy variables are identified by adding a D to the definitions in the preceding list.

We first estimated a continuous permanent market wage from the available information. To accomplish this, we selected two groups from households in which the head's age was between 25 and 64. This step does not apply to post-age 65 retired families. The two groups consist of (1) families in which only a male adult currently works full-time and (2) families in which only a female adult currently works full time.

For each group,

$$Y^* = f(EY_i^*, NEY^*) \tag{A.4}$$

$i = m$ or f, and $Y^* =$ permanent earned and nonearned income of the family.

A regression was estimated for each of the two groups with measured income as the dependent variable and the independent variables included determinants of EY_i^* and a binary variable for NEY^* ($NEYSD$) that took the value one if the family received income from any of the sources in Equation A.3.

Determinants of EY_i^* in our work were:

Years of schooling	= EDUC
Experience and experience squared	= EXP, EXP2
Has pain "very often" or "fairly often"	= PAIN
Black	= BLACK
Spanish surname	= SURNAME
NonEnglish.language spoken at home when a child	= NONENG
Catholic	= CATH
Protestant	= PROT
Population of Primary Sampling Unit	= POP
Northeast Census Area	= NE
South Census Area	= S
West Census Area	= W

To permit structural differences in wage determination among persons with varying amounts of schooling, the two groups were further subdivided into educational attainment groups for estimation purposes: less than nine years; nine to twelve years; and thirteen and over years of schooling. The experience variable was derived on the basis of the respondent's age and educational attainment. It was assumed that persons with more schooling enter the labor force later.[1] The experience variable accounts for periods of nonparticipation after the individual first enters the workforce. Such absences do not present a serious problem for males and females who are sole "breadwinners," as they tend to remain in the labor force on a rather continuous basis.[2] However, in a later step, we used the parameter estimates obtained from this regression to project EY^* for persons who are *not* sole breadwinners as well as those who are. Labor force participation of married women is notably noncontinuous, and experience variables, such as ours, are somewhat inaccurate for some of these persons. In view of the complexity of the analysis in subsequent steps, we decided early in our analysis to follow a policy of "benign neglect" on this issue; our study shares this deficiency with the vast majority of wage-determination studies.

Since CATH and PROT identify Catholics and Protestants, the omitted category includes Jews, persons with nonWestern religions, and those without a religious preference. We included a binary variable identifying Jewish respondents in initial regressions, but the sample sizes on this variable in some of the six regressions were too small. Given NE, S, and W, the omitted Census Area is North Central. Given the parameter estimates as presented in the following sections, a predicted hourly wage for every adult in the sample was calculated by dividing predicted EY_m and EY_f by 2,000 hours (fifty weeks times forty hours per week).

With estimates of EY_m* and EY_f*, we derived a continuous estimate of permanent nonemployment income (NEY*) as a second step. In the first step, we restricted the regression analysis to households with one full-time breadwinner for two reasons. First, we deemed it desirable to include only one set of wage determinant variables in the regression rather than separate sets for adult males and females. Second, we wanted to exclude any effects the explanatory variables might have on work hours. Our method in the first stage required us to assume that the wage determination structure does not differ systematically according to family type or size. Although this assumption is somewhat tenable for earned income, it has no basis whatsoever for nonearned income, since transfer programs use family structure as a central criterion for establishing eligibility and the size of payments. Therefore, for purposes of the remaining steps, we stratified the samples on the same basis as in the access regressions reported in chapters 5 and 6: female heads of households aged 25 to 64; married men aged 25 to 64; married women aged 25 to 64; and two-person families in which both husband and wife are retired and both are over age 65. Since the retirees, by definition, had no earned income in 1974, these families entered the analysis here for the first time.

Given estimates of permanent earned income, EY_m and EY_f, equation A.4 may be rewritten as

$$Y = EY_m* - EY_f* = NEY* + NEY\dagger + R \qquad (A.5)$$

where $NEY\dagger$ represents transfer payments from "transitory" sources identified by the Medical Access Study and R is a composite of a random error, influences related to variables such as ability that are omitted from the wage-generating equations, and transitory income not included in $NEY\dagger$.

$$NEY\dagger = SSI + FR + UC + WC + PA \qquad (A.6)$$

To generate an estimate of NEY* and the remaining nonemployment income $NEY\dagger$, we regressed the left side of equation A.5 on dummy variables INTDIVD through VAD for NEY* and SSID through PAD for $NEY\dagger$. The coefficients estimated from this regression represent mean nonemployment income flow from *each* source identified by the Medical Access Study. Since we stratified on the basis of household demographic status, we preserved important intergroup variation among these means.

Having estimated the nonemployment income regressions, we then proceeded to the third step and estimated shadow wages. As we noted in chapter 1, on theoretical grounds, the shadow wage equals the market wage for employed persons. For the nonemployed, the shadow wage exceeds the market wage for employed persons. For the nonemployed, the shadow wage exceeds the market wage. An approximation of the shadow wage for the nonemployed may be obtained from an estimated labor supply function evaluated at zero hours of work.

For illustrative purposes, we can assume the following linear supply curve:

$$H = \alpha_0 + \alpha_1 W_s + \alpha_2 Z \qquad (A.7)$$

where H is the number of workhours supplied to the market, W_s is the shadow wage and Z is any exogenous shift variable relevant to the supply curve. To derive the shadow wage for the nonemployed, one may set $H = 0$. Then,

$$W_s = \frac{\alpha_0 + \alpha_2 Z}{\alpha_1} \qquad (A.8)$$

Equation A.8 is the intercept of the traditional labor supply curve. For $H > 0$, the shadow and market wages are equal theoretically. They will never be the same in a research setting since market wages are observed directly, while home wages are derived from an estimated supply equation that reflects average responses of individuals in the sample. Economic theory provides no guide for choosing between these two alternatives.[3] For persons who have lost their jobs during recessions, the home wage may be calculated at $H = 0$, or at $H =$ some small positive number if one wants to account for time the unemployed spend in job search. Our methodology assumes that the shadow wage calculated in this manner is a reasonable estimate of an individual's time price. This notion is subject to some questions if people have preferences about the ways they spend their time.

There are, in the literature, several reviews of recent econometric studies of labor supply.[4] Unfortunately, they reveal a wide degree of dispersion in estimated parameters, and we therefore have been reluctant to use the results of any past study for our purposes. Moreover, data on some of the explanatory variables of previous studies are not available on the MAS, and this information would be necessary for purposes of projecting home wages.

For these reasons, we have estimated labor supply functions for married males, married females, and unmarried female heads using MAS data. This data base does not provide a continuous estimate of work hours, but information on current employment status allows one to distinguish among full-time, part-time, and nonemployed individuals. Assuming that full-time employees work forty hours weekly, we estimated labor supply equations using two-limit probit analysis (TLP) and ordinary least squares (OLS). TLP is preferable because of the concentration of values of the dependent variable at forty hours, an upper bound, and zero hours, a lower bound. Rosett and Nelson compared estimated TLP parameters when the values of the nonlimit or intermediate values are known and when one only knows that the observation falls between the upper (in our application, forty hours) and lower limit (here, zero hours).[5] They found the parameters based on no knowledge of intermediate values to be reasonably close to the parameters based on knowledge of nonlimit *and* limit values. Since we know only that part-time work part-time, their findings are particularly encouraging.

Explanatory variables in the labor supply regressions for married persons were:

Hourly wage of household head	= HDY
Hourly wage of spouse	= SPY
Permanent non-employment income	= NEYP
Other non-employment income (NEY† + R)	= RESIDF
Head has pain "very often," "fairly often"	= HDPAIN (in regressions on heads)
Spouse has pain "very often," "fairly often"	= SPPAIN (in regressions on spouses)
Head is black	= BLACK
Head has Spanish surname	= SURNAME
Head age 25–30 (spouse age 25–30)	= HD1 (SP1)
Head age 31–40 (spouse age 31–40)	= HD2 (SP2)
Head age 41–50 (spouse age 41–50)	= HD3 (SP3)
Number of children in household under age 2	= CHILD1
Number of children in household ages 2–5	= CHILD2
Number of children in household ages 6–15	= CHILD3
Number of children in household ages 16–19	= CHILD4
Number of adults in household other than head or spouse ages 20–64	= ADULT1
Number of adults in household other than head or spouse ages 65 and over	= ADULT2

The unmarried female regressions only contain a household head wage. Since the post-65 group is limited to retirees, labor supply analysis is inapplicable.

In summary, our procedure allowed us to estimate market wages, permanent and transitory-residual nonearned income, and shadow wages from a single family income measure. Clearly these estimates are based on a number of underlying assumptions, and more direct estimates would have been more desirable. However, we had no choice.

Empirical Results

Family Income Regressions for Generating Permanent Earnings

Our first step involved estimating regressions on full-time employed, single bread-winner adults between the ages 25 and 64 with measured family income as the dependent variable to derive estimates of permanent earnings for men and women. We estimated six regressions (three educational attainment groups by sex). The principal results are reflected in table A–1.

The regressions are much more successful in explaining male than female family income. In the male regressions, schooling, experience, and race-ethnicity, as judged by the coefficients of BLACK and SURNAME, have anticipated impacts on income and their associated coefficients are frequently statistically significant. The estimated parameters on the schooling variable clearly indicate that the marginal impact of an additional year of schooling is higher at higher levels of educational attainment. Experience has a greater effect on income in the thirteen plus schooling group initially, but income peaks earlier too (27.1 years for the thirteen plus group versus 29.6 years for the eight and under group, and 29.8 years for the nine-twelve group). There are no systematic regional or city-size effects. This result is not too surprising since all monetarily-expressed variables have been deflated by an area price index prior to estimation.[6]

Although the results for females are more erratic, it is essential to consider that the regressions are designed to account for income variation *within* the three educational attainment groups. As the mean values for family income variables indicate, there is substantial variation in family income among the three educational groups.[7] Our measures of predicted permanent earnings, based on all coefficients except the permanent nonemployment variable, preserve these differences.

Nonearned Income Regressions

In the second step, we regressed the difference between family income and estimated permanent earned income on a set of binary variables representing

Table A-1
Family Income Regressions

Variable	Males, Age in Years			Females, Age in Years		
	0-8	9-12	13+	0-8	9-12	13+
EDUC	426.3† (204.9)	1273.1* (412.4)	1610.4* (374.0)	-330.9 (269.2)	364.8 (720.0)	777.6 (549.9)
EXP	265.5 (215.6)	259.1 (151.0)	666.3* (207.4)	555.7 (312.4)	435.1 (291.8)	-27.3 (259.6)
EXP2	-4.48 (3.40)	-3.26 (3.09)	-12.30† (5.93)	-9.89† (4.59)	-8.97 (5.86)	2.67 (6.54)
PAIN	-1034.7 (1277.3)	-1452.6 (1201.9)	-53.8 (2043.4)	-1639.0 (1055.0)	435.2 (1876.5)	-1225.0 (1717.3)
BLACK	-1204.2 (1320.6)	-1872.7 (1341.4)	-5210.0* (2589.2)	-113.7 (1427.8)	230.7 (1810.6)	127.7 (2246.8)
SURNAME	-4427.2† (1913.4)	-3039.2† (1376.5)	-63.2 (2881.2)	-1681.9 (1969.4)	-1597.6 (3264.3)	2571.4 (4915.8)
NONENG	-2297.0 (2016.4)	617.2 (992.7)	-2563.3 (1419.1)	-2998.5 (1783.0)	-45.6 (1932.6)	2310.6 (1926.1)
CATH	4940.9† (2012.9)	-566.1 (1455.6)	-4555.7* (1712.3)	1483.6 (1667.0)	-907.6 (2761.8)	-1906.3 (2524.8)
PROT	1088.0 (1691.4)	-1337.3 (1315.1)	-5622.6* (1623.6)	(—)	-3589.4 (2446.2)	838.7 (2114.9)
POP	47.8 (54.9)	63.5 (43.0)	67.5 (64.0)	110.0 (73.2)	-84.3 (76.4)	0.82 (81.75)
NE	-1866.8 (1578.2)	-2432.7† (1126.9)	-1256.0 (1571.3)	1656.1 (1910.1)	-2135.7 (2252.7)	-1023.2 (2351.6)
S	-3142.0† (1253.6)	-95.5 (992.7)	3285.2† (1646.1)	-1758.6 (1443.1)	-3180.5 (1906.5)	1227.4 (2128.8)

WEST	1489.7 (1924.8)	−1053.5 (1585.5)	3186.0 (1958.7)	−1839.3 (2139.0)	722.2 (2016.1)
NEY	952.8 (914.2)	3716.7* (860.3)	2963.0* (924.0)	2505.5† (1108.6)	1180.2 (948.3)
	$R^2 = 0.30$ $F_{(15,126)} = 3.6*$	$R^2 = 0.27$ $F_{(15,306)} = 7.6*$	$R^2 = 0.44$ $F_{(14,44)} = 2.5$	$R^2 = 0.10$ $F_{(15,152)} = 1.1$	$R^2 = 0.11$ $F_{(15,100)} = 0.8$

*Significant at 1 percent level; †significant at 5 percent level.

sources of nonearned income. For retirees, all family income is from such sources, and hence measured family income and nonearned income coincide.

An issue that must be resolved in the process of implementing the second step is the treatment of the permanent earnings of part-time and nonemployed workers. The MAS reveals current employment status. However, current employment status is subject to change, especially during recessionary periods. For purposes of the regression analysis, we would have preferred to have an indicator of usual employment status (such as is available from the Health Interview Survey analyzed in chapter 4). We did experiment with alternative ways of treating employment status. In one variant, all heads and spouses were assumed to work 2,000 hours annually. In a second variant, current employment status was assumed to be the usual status and part-timers were assumed to work 1,000 hours and nonemployed persons, zero hours. Although the level of the dependent variable was greatly affected by the specific assumptions made, the parameter estimates of the nonearned income regressions proved to be reasonably insensitive to the variant chosen. Our empirical results for step two, based on the second variant, are presented in table A-2.

It is useful to consider permanent (NEY^*) and transitory ($NEY\dagger$) sources separately when evaluating these results. Not surprisingly, the statistically significant coefficients with anticipated positive signs tend to refer to components of NEY^*. Among these, the most important are INTDIVD (= interest and dividend income) and PPD (= private pension income). The coefficient on RENTD (= rental income) is statistically significant for married households, but not for the other two groups. A negative bias is introduced into the coefficients of the $NEY\dagger$ variable because payment is largely contingent on income losses from other sources, but these payments tend to be smaller than the losses. This tendency is even more apparent when all adults in the sample are assumed to usually work full-time.

Two income measures have been derived from the estimated parameters of the first, second, and fourth regressions presented in table A-2. The first is an estimate of NEY^*. The second is a variable termed RESID, which includes $NEY\dagger$ and these regressions' results.

Labor Supply Regressions for Generating Shadow Wages

In step 3, we estimated hourly earnings and nonearned income obtained from the first two steps to enter as explanatory variables in a labor supply regression. Parameters estimated from these regressions can be used to calculate shadow wages for nonemployed and employed adults. An earlier study by Cogan presented rather encouraging evidence, suggesting that "reasonable" shadow wages can be calculated by this approach.[8] Our own experience does not support this view. Although our estimated labor supply equations are quite plausible, the predicted shadow wages frequently are quite implausible, necessitating a somewhat different approach in our analysis of access in chapters 5 and 6.

Table A-2
Nonearned Income Regressions

Variable	Married Households Ages 25–64	Unmarried Female Heads Ages 25–64	Retirees Ages 65 and over	
INDIVD	3652.1*	2595.4*	4934.1*	5151.1*
	(483.2)	(957.0)	(810.7)	(802.2)
RENTD	2333.9*	1915.1	−223.7	−72.0
	(830.0)	(1635.2)	(1286.1)	(1289.0)
SSRD	3876.9*	2555.4	856.0	−2348.0
	(1381.1)	(1598.6)	(2519.1)	(1592.0)
SSSD	1492.2	2770.4†	7311.4†	−
	(2198.0)	(1091.4)	(3447.3)	(−)
PPD	5661.7*	4290.0†	2156.7*	2059.2*
	(1149.3)	(1697.2)	(753.8)	(774.5)
ACSD	−1426.3	1904.6†	−	−
	(1918.0)	(955.3)	(−)	(−)
AFAD	−705.7	−	−	−
	(1605.8)	(−)	(−)	(−)
VAD	612.7	−	920.5	992.4
	(1012.9)	(−)	(1392.3)	(1402.7)
UCD	−647.1	1331.6	−	−
	(741.8)	(1629.4)	(−)	(−)
WCD	982.1	240.2	−	−
	(1874.1)	(2853.3)	(−)	(−)
PAD	30.1	1434.7	−129.8	−
	(1512.8)	(829.1)	(2344.7)	(−)
SSID	−33.9	885.5	−415.7	−1613.5
	(1933.5)	(1741.7)	(1948.1)	(1783.4)
FRIENDD	−539.0	−3161.0	1162.2	−
	(1401.8)	(1741.6)	(2364.2)	(−)
OTHD	−2146.2	−	−	−
	(2776.3)	(−)	(−)	(−)
CONSTANT			3246.1	6461.7
	(−)	(−)	(−)	(−)
	$R^2 = 0.07$	$R^2 = 0.08$	$R^2 = 0.30$	$R^2 = 0.27$
	$F(14,1776) =$	$F(12,457) =$	$F(9,155) =$	$F(6,158) =$
	9.3*	3.3*	7.4*	9.9*

*Significant at the 1 percent level; †significant at the 5 percent level.

Estimated labor supply equations are presented in table A-3. Both two-limit probit (TLP) and ordinary least squares (OLS) estimates are presented. The natural logarithms of the hourly wage terms (LHDY and LSPY) have been substituted for the linear wage terms (HDY and SPY) in the regressions contained in table A-3. We made this substitution after obtaining negative predicted home wages with linear wages HDY and SPY as explanatory variables. Negative shadow wages are fully inconsistent with the underlying theory. Cogan used the log of

Table A-3
Hours Regressions

| | Married Households Ages 25-64 | | | | Unmarried Female Heads Ages 25-64 | |
| | Male | | Female | | | |
	TLP	OLS	TLP	OLS	TLP	OLS
LHDY	32.36† (15.08)	1.27 (0.67)	-20.55 (10.85)	-2.53 (1.43)	23.14 (16.54)	1.49 (1.84)
LSPY	-3.42 (10.31)	0.34 (0.38)	1.55 (6.24)	1.89 (0.83)	— (—)	— (—)
NEYP	-0.013* (0.002)	-0.0010* (0.001)	-0.0027 (0.0013)	-0.0003 (0.0002)	-0.015* (0.004)	-0.002* (0.0004)
RESID	-0.004* (0.0007)	-0.0002* (0.00003)	-0.0087* (0.0006)	-0.0012* (0.00007)	-0.012* (0.0002)	-0.001* (0.0002)
HDPAIN	-16.04 (14.38)	-1.46 (0.76)	— (—)	— (—)	33.94† (14.25)	-3.79† (1.56)
SPPAIN	— (—)	— (—)	-21.15† (10.60)	-2.54 (1.40)	— (—)	— (—)
BLACK	-49.47* (13.23)	-2.63* (0.67)	49.26* (10.72)	7.06* (1.46)	5.83 (17.07)	0.64 (1.82)
SURNAME	-11.85 (14.53)	-0.20 (0.67)	-2.74 (11.09)	-0.31 (1.36)	-48.57† (19.71)	-6.36* (2.24)
HD1	172.13* (21.08)	14.81* (0.92)	— (—)	— (—)	132.22* (28.61)	13.88* (2.24)
HD2	140.49* (15.77)	14.10 (0.84)	— (—)	— (—)	126.25* (27.50)	13.63* (2.92)
HD3	124.86* (14.72)	13.38 (0.82)	— (—)	— (—)	58.47* (24.73)	7.52* (2.81)
HD4	76.82* (12.36)	10.96 (0.81)	— (—)	— (—)	43.55* (23.47)	5.38† (2.67)

	(1)	(2)	(3)	(4)	(5)	(6)
SP1	— (—)	— (—)	101.08* (19.35)	14.06* (2.54)	— (—)	— (—)
SP2	— (—)	— (—)	85.69* (18.97)	12.10* (2.50)	— (—)	— (—)
SP3	— (—)	— (—)	63.36* (18.59)	9.20* (2.46)	— (—)	— (—)
SP4	— (—)	— (—)	20.85 (18.99)	3.25 (2.44)	— (—)	— (—)
CHILD1	-4.61 (15.51)	-0.12 (0.55)	-49.47* (9.43)	-6.54* (1.21)	-74.99* (28.41)	-9.24* (3.15)
CHILD2	-2.33 (9.01)	0.13 (0.34)	-47.06* (6.07)	-5.93* (0.76)	-66.30* (17.12)	-8.03* (1.90)
CHILD3	-3.02* (0.41)	-0.11 (0.17)	-8.54* (2.77)	-1.21* (0.37)	-24.04* (6.42)	-2.66* (0.73)
CHILD4	13.45 (8.63)	0.64 (0.34)	-0.85 (5.39)	0.15 (0.73)	5.63* (1.47)	-0.47 (1.56)
ADULT1	-2.32 (9.34)	-0.03 (0.46)	11.83 (7.63)	1.63 (1.02)	12.72 (15.83)	-1.08 (1.78)
ADULT2	48.08 (31.68)	2.64 (1.29)	-1.40 (20.76)	-0.84 (2.79)	59.50* (39.08)	7.62 (4.16)
CONS	17.23* (0.30)	23.20 (—)	-34.42 (26.28)	10.81 (—)	42.19 (34.11)	25.08 (—)
σ	76.91	$R^2 = 0.31$	91.06	$R^2 = 0.26$	91.19	$R^2 = 0.36$
	$F_{(17,1670)} = 44.38^*$		$F_{(17,1670)} = 33.74^*$		$F_{(16,3971)} = 14.04^*$	

*Significant at 1 percent level; †significant at 5 percent level.

wages, and, on reflection, with good reason. One is unlikely to obtain positive shadow wages with a linear specification of the wage component.

On the whole, the labor supply results are quite plausible. Moreover, the results compare very favorably to those from labor supply studies for which more direct measures of the financial variables were available. The "own" wage effects, reflected by the coefficient of LHDY in the first, second, fifth, and sixth regressions and the coefficient of LSPY in the third and fourth, are positive—implying a positively sloped labor supply curve. This result implies in turn that as work hours decline, as a consequence of job loss, for example, the individual lowers the value he attributes to his own time. The cross-wage effects, reflected by the coefficient of LSPY in the first and second regressions and the coefficient of LHDY in the third and fourth, are negative in three out of the four married person regressions. The notion does not apply, of course, in the (unmarried) female head regressions. This result can be shown to imply that, on the average, the shadow wage is higher for persons who have spouses with a high earnings potential.

The coefficients on the two nonemployment income variables, NEYP and RESID, are uniformly negative and statistically significant in the majority of regressions. Not surprisingly, the permanent income coefficients tend to be larger in absolute terms than their transitory-residual income counterparts. Translated into shadow wages, these results imply that families with higher levels of nonearned income have higher shadow wages.

The estimated age parameters (HD1 through HD4 and SP1 through SP4) indicate that the supply of labor curve shifts upward with age (in other words, there is less labor supplied). Equivalently, the shadow wage rises. The CHILD coefficients imply that mothers of small children work less; these variables essentially demonstrate no impact on the work patterns of males. This result is fully consistent with past evidence.[9]

The BLACK and SURNAME coefficients reveal a mixed result. For blacks, the regressions suggest that black men work less and black women more, holding all other factors constant. The coefficients are consistently negative for Spanish-surnamed individuals, but are only statistically significant in the unmarried female head regressions.

The remaining variables, which pertain to health (HDPAIN and SPPAIN) and the presence of adults other than the head and spouse in the household (ADULT1 and ADULT2), show essentially no effect.

The partial effects of the model's explanatory variables on the shadow wage are summarized in table A-4. While the coefficients tend to be quite plausible, extensive efforts to derive reasonable predicted shadow wages from these regressions proved to be fruitless. Reasonable means can sometimes be obtained, but the variances about the means are always implausibly high, that is, coefficients of variation of 10 and more. Comparing our results with Cogan's, it is evident that Cogan's mean predicted shadow wages are plausible, but Cogan presented

Table A-4
Effects of Exogenous Variables on the Shadow Wage

Variable	Males	Married Females	Unmarried Females
Cross-wage	Unclear	Positive	Inapplicable
Permanent nonearned income	Positive	Almost zero	Positive
Transitory-residual nonearned income	Positive	Positive	Positive
Age	Positive	Positive	Positive
Young children	Almost zero	Positive	Positive
Older children	Almost zero	Positive to zero	Positive to zero
Race-ethnicity:			
black	Positive	Negative	Almost zero
Spanish surname	Positive	Negative	Almost zero
Poor health	Almost zero	Almost zero	Almost zero
Other adults	Almost zero	Almost zero	Almost zero

no evidence as dispersion of shadow wages. To the extent that the dispersion is overstated by this approach, errors-in-variables are introduced when the predicted shadow wage is an explanatory variable, as in the access regressions presented in chapters 5 and 6; and, given the standard assumptions that economists make under such circumstances, the resulting parameter estimates are biased toward zero.

As we have noted, the market wage provides an appropriate measure of the time price for employed persons. For nonemployed persons, the home wage exceeds the market wage. This would imply at first glance that the predicted market wage is too low. Another explanation, especially in the case of the unemployed, is that the person's market wage is temporarily depressed. If so, the predicted market wage, which after all does not take temporary factors into account, would overstate the market wage. In view of the dispersion problem and preliminary access regressions, it appears that the predicted market wage provides a better estimate of the time price of employed persons than the predicted shadow wage. Our adjustment for the nonemployed has been described in chapter 5.

Notes

1. Our method for defining experience and experience-squared followed Paul T. Schultz, *Estimating Labor Supply Functions for Married Women,* Santa Monica, California: Rand Corporation (R-1265-NIH/EDA), 1975.

2. William G. Bowen and T. Aldrich Finegan, *The Economics of Labor Force Participation,* Princeton, New Jersey: Princeton University Press, 1969;

Frank Sloan and Somchai Richupan, "Short-Run Supply Responses of Professional Nurses: A Microanalysis," *Journal of Human Resources* X (Spring):241–257, 1975.

3. We shall discuss this point more fully below.

4. Glen G. Cain and Harold Watts (eds.), *Income Maintenance and Labor Supply: Econometric Studies,* Chicago: Markham Press, 1973.

5. Richard N. Rosett and Forrest D. Nelson, "Estimation of the Two-Limit Probit Regression Model." *Econometrica* 43 (January): 140–146, 1975.

6. See Bruce Steinwald and Frank Sloan, "Determinants of Physicians' Fees," *Journal of Business* 47 (October):493–511, 1974, for a description of this index.

7. Means and standard deviations of variables included in this appendix's regressions are available from the authors on request.

8. John F. Cogan, *Labor Supply and the Value of the Housewife's Time,* Santa Monica, California: Rand Corporation (R-1461-OEO/EDA/RF), 1975.

9. See, for example, Solomon W. Polachek. "Potential Biases in Measuring Male-Female Discrimination," *Journal of Human Resources* X (Spring):205–229, 1975.

Index

Access measures, 3–6, 39, 73–78, 90, 97
Activity limitation categories, 82–83, 89, 91
Acton, Jan Paul, 30–32
Aday, Lu Ann, 76
Aid to Families with Dependent Children (AFDC), 7, 151
"Amenities," 24, 36, 51, 79, 97, 99, 143, 144, 145
Andersen, Ronald, 4, 26–27, 76
Appointment delays, 30, 36–38, 95, 131, 142–143, 145–146, 148–149, 152
Asset-debt composition of households, 9–11
Autocorrelation, 57–58, 63, 71

Bach, George L., 9–11
Becker, Gary S., 99
Bed-disability days, 46, 49, 56, 58, 63, 67, 70, 148, 150
Benham, Lee and Alexandra, 28–29
Bentkover, Judith D., 49
Berry, Charles, 83
Blendon, Robert J., 28
Bobula, Joel D., 131
Brenner, M. Harvey, xvii, 19, 55, 67, 69, 149

Canada: universal health insurance, 33–35
Care, continuity of, 79, 88–89, 150
Central cities, 83, 89, 92
Children, 28, 29, 46, 47, 49, 50, 63, 69
Chronic illness, 82–83
Classification functions, 106–108
Community size variables, 83, 89
Consumer demand, 11–12, 16, 18, 99–100, 101
Creditor-debtor account, 9–11
Cromwell, Jerry, 127

Cross-sectional analysis, 27, 28–29, 35–38, 149
  years 1969–1975, 46–54
  year 1974, 73–78, 90
Cyclical/secular trends, 45, 46, 49, 51, 54, 69, 149

Darby, Michael R., 16
Davis, Karen, 12–13
Demand models, 26–27
"Discouraged worker effects," 21
Discriminate analysis, 96, 102, 106–108, 150
Durbin-Watson statistics, 57–58, 63

Economic efficiency, 21
Economic Stabilization Program (ESP), 131–132, 143–144
Economy theory of the household, 99–101
Education variable, 81–82, 88, 89, 90, 91, 150
Eisenberg, Barry S., 131
Elderly, 11, 13, 35, 50, 82, 86
  visit rates, 28, 46, 47, 63, 69
Emergency room care, 50, 51, 54, 69, 95, 96, 115, 118, 151
Employment status
  and access measures, 77–78, 79–80, 89, 90, 135
  and explanatory variables, 80–86, 88
  and utilization, 51–54, 149
Enabling factors, 27, 54, 82
Endogenous/exogenous variables, 26, 56–57, 67, 98–99
Enterline, Philip E., 33–34
Equality-in-use standard, 5
Equilibrium, price-output, 23
Explanatory variables, 26–27, 80–86

Family size, 47–49, 81, 105, 119, 139
Farms, 83, 89

171

About the Authors

Frank A. Sloan is professor, Department of Economics, and senior research associate, Institute for Public Policy Studies, Vanderbilt University. He received the B.A. from Oberlin College and the Ph.D. in economics from Harvard University. He was a summer intern on the President's Council of Economic Advisors, a Woodrow Wilson National Fellow, and has served as research associate with the Rand Corporation, lecturer at the Department of Economics, University of California at Los Angeles, and associate professor at the Department of Economics, University of Florida. He serves as a consultant to a number of government and private organizations. Dr. Sloan is coauthor of *Private Physicians and Public Programs* (Lexington Books, 1978).

Judith D. Bentkover is a senior health economist at Arthur D. Little, Inc. She received the B.A. from Douglass College of Rutgers University and the Ph.D. in Economics from Tufts University. Her research includes several federal, state, and local projects involving modeling, analysis, and policy evaluation in the area of applied microeconomics. Dr. Bentkover is also a part-time faculty member at Simmons College in Boston, Massachusetts.